FANTASTIC FACTS
THE BODY

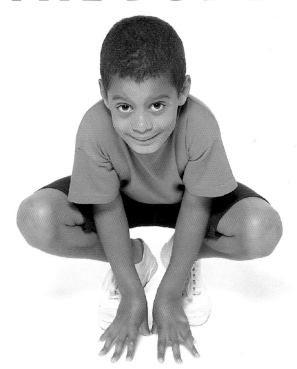

STEPHEN PARKER

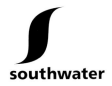

southwater

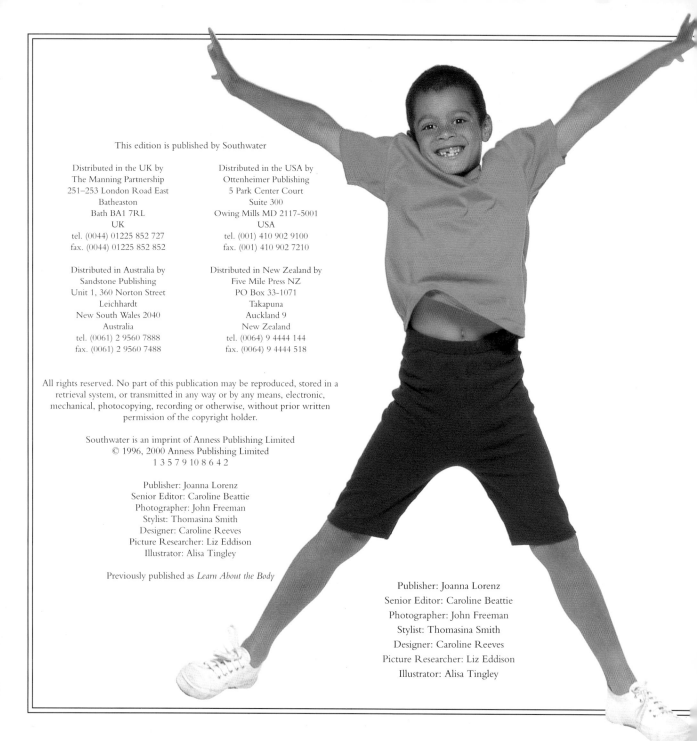

This edition is published by Southwater

Distributed in the UK by
The Manning Partnership
251–253 London Road East
Batheaston
Bath BA1 7RL
UK
tel. (0044) 01225 852 727
fax. (0044) 01225 852 852

Distributed in the USA by
Ottenheimer Publishing
5 Park Center Court
Suite 300
Owing Mills MD 2117-5001
USA
tel. (001) 410 902 9100
fax. (001) 410 902 7210

Distributed in Australia by
Sandstone Publishing
Unit 1, 360 Norton Street
Leichhardt
New South Wales 2040
Australia
tel. (0061) 2 9560 7888
fax. (0061) 2 9560 7488

Distributed in New Zealand by
Five Mile Press NZ
PO Box 33-1071
Takapuna
Auckland 9
New Zealand
tel. (0064) 9 4444 144
fax. (0064) 9 4444 518

Southwater is an imprint of Anness Publishing Limited
© 1996, 2000 Anness Publishing Limited
1 3 5 7 9 10 8 6 4 2

Publisher: Joanna Lorenz
Senior Editor: Caroline Beattie
Photographer: John Freeman
Stylist: Thomasina Smith
Designer: Caroline Reeves
Picture Researcher: Liz Eddison
Illustrator: Alisa Tingley

Previously published as Learn About the Body

Publisher: Joanna Lorenz
Senior Editor: Caroline Beattie
Photographer: John Freeman
Stylist: Thomasina Smith
Designer: Caroline Reeves
Picture Researcher: Liz Eddison
Illustrator: Alisa Tingley

THE BODY

CONTENTS

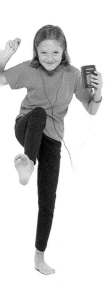

YOUR BODY

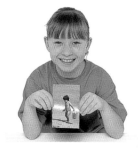

Bodies change through their lives. They grow bigger, then after many years, they may shrink slightly smaller. Can you remember how small you were, and how big and tall everyone else seemed, when you were a baby? What are your earliest memories?

WHAT do you see most each day? Schoolwork, perhaps? Or television? Most people spend a long time each day looking at bodies – human bodies belonging to family, friends, teachers, relatives, store owners and many other people. You watch these bodies move around, walk and talk, eat, laugh, cry and carry out their daily lives. You probably know a lot about the people you see every day. But how much do you know about their bodies – and about your own body? Why does the human body have two arms and two legs, with the head on top? Why does it have hair and fingernails? How does it run, jump and speak? What happens to food after it is swallowed? And how does the body work inside?

The body has a strong framework of bones, to hold it up. There are more than 200 bones inside the body, and hundreds of other parts, too.

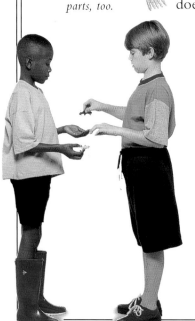

Different types

There are two main kinds of human body: male and female. The female ones are called girls when young and women when grown-up. The male ones are called boys when young and men when grown-up.

Different shapes

Bodies vary on the outside, even when they are all the same age. Some are taller than others. Some have slightly different colored hair, eyes and skin. But on the inside, bodies are all much the same.

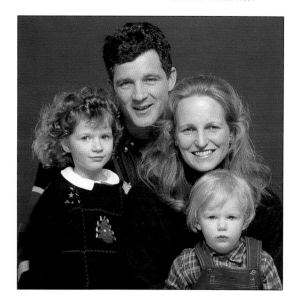

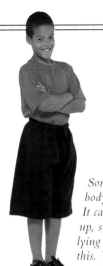

Sometimes the body needs to eat. Food gives it energy and nutrients, for moving around, growing and carrying out all its living processes.

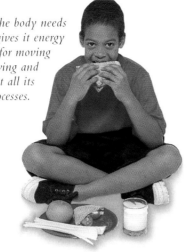

Sometimes the body stays still. It can be standing up, sitting down or lying when it does this. Yet inside, parts like the heart are still moving.

Sometimes the body does active things, like running. It can jog slowly or sprint fast, and kick or throw a ball at the same time!

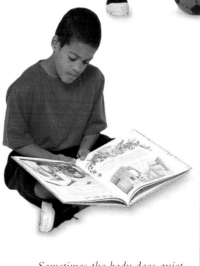

This book answers all these questions, and many more. It shows how your eyes work, what your bones look like, how your heart beats, and what happens in your brain. Learning about the body is easy, because you always have one to study!

FACT BOX

• Each human body is a member of the animal group, or species, that scientists call *Homo sapiens* ("Wise Human").

• There are about 5,700 million human bodies in the world. This compares with approximately 1,200 million sheep, and 500 million dogs.

• No animals have spread to as many places in the world as us. People live in snowy polar lands, in tropical forests, in arid deserts and on high mountains. After us, the next most widespread animal is the house mouse.

Sometimes the body rests and sleeps. Every body needs to sleep, usually at night. Younger bodies generally need more sleep than older ones.

Sometimes the body does quiet things, like reading, listening to music, drawing pictures or solving puzzles. It can learn lots of new skills and information at this time.

MEASURE YOUR BODY

To measure your weight, simply stand on a scale. Take off your shoes and heavy clothing, like your coat and sweater, since these make you seem heavier. Don't worry about light clothing like T-shirts. Note your weight in pounds.

How tall are you? How much do you weigh? What size shoes do you take? You may know the answers to these questions – or you can find out by measuring. But what about your hat, collar or glove size? You can measure the body to find out its size and shape, for many reasons. A doctor measures the weight of a new baby to make sure it is healthy and growing well. An optician measures a person's eyes, for glasses. A tailor measures neck, waist, chest, arms and legs, to make well-fitting clothes. How do you measure up?

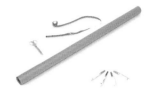

You will need: tape measure, large roll of paper (such as the back of a roll of unwanted wallpaper), colored pens, scissors.

Draw a graph of your body measurements over months, or even years.

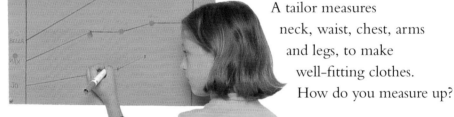

Measure parts of your body

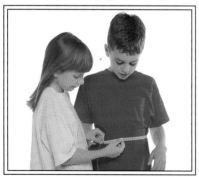

1 Measure around the waist at the level where you'd wear a belt.

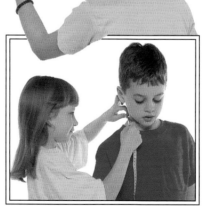

2 Measure around the neck, at its narrowest point.

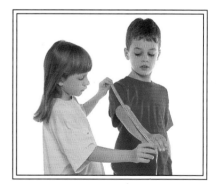

3 Measure the arm from the point of the shoulder to the wrist.

You could make a chart of your body's different measurements over the years. Use different colors on the graph for height, weight, waist size and so on. Measure yourself at regular times, such as every three months, or on your birthday, or on the last day of each school term. Which measurement changes most, and which alters least?

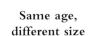

Same age, different size

Get together with some friends of the same age (in years). How much variation is there between you all in height or weight? Try the same test on children who are much younger, such as two years old. Do the same for grown-ups who are 20 years old. Which age has most variation?

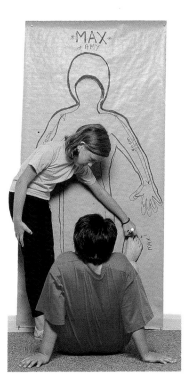

Body outline

Trace around the whole body with a colored pen. Trace around friends, too. Label each tracing with the date. Next time, use different colored pens. Who's grown the most?

Feet and hands

Draw carefully around your foot and hand. Do the same for friends. Who has the thinnest fingers, the widest palm or the thickest wrist?

FACES

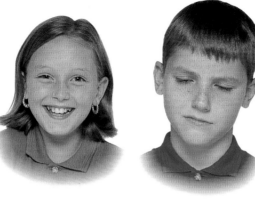

Face paints or cosmetic makeup can alter a face completely. You can become a funny clown, a wizened witch or a movie star. Makeup also helps with acting and pretending. If it makes you look like an animal, such as a cat or mouse, you may find it easier to act like that animal.

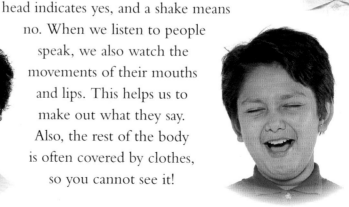

LOOK in the mirror. Which part of your body do you see? Probably, your face. This is the most-looked-at part of anybody's body, for many reasons. Faces are truly fascinating. They show people's moods – happy, sad, pleased, worried, tired or thoughtful. Tiny movements of the eyebrows and eyelids can mean a lot, like surprise or anger. A flicker around the lips may mean that a smile is coming, or a frown. In most countries a nod of the head indicates yes, and a shake means no. When we listen to people speak, we also watch the movements of their mouths and lips. This helps us to make out what they say. Also, the rest of the body is often covered by clothes, so you cannot see it!

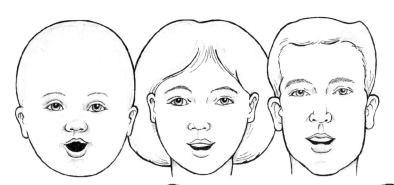

How faces change with age

As you grow, your face gets bigger. It also changes its proportions. A baby's face is small compared to the size of its whole head. Its eyes and forehead are big, its nose and mouth are small. In a grown-up, the nose and mouth take up more of the face. And the face takes up more than half of the front of the head.

Two-sided face

Both sides of a face look the same. They could be perfect mirror images of each other. But are they exactly identical – that is, are they symmetrical? Here is a normal photograph of a boy. Compare it with the following faces.

Two right sides

The left side of this photograph has been cut away, and replaced with a reversed version of the right side. So this face is the boy's right half plus a mirror image of it. Does it look like the real face, which is shown on the left?

Two left sides

In this version, the right side of the photograph is replaced by a reversed version of the left side. So this shows the face's left half plus a mirror-image of it. Does it look more like the real face than the two-right-sides one on the left?

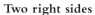

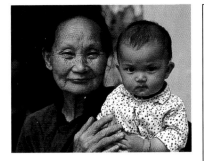

Young and old

A baby's face usually has smooth, soft skin. After many years, the skin may develop wrinkles and lines. This is entirely natural. It is more likely to happen if the person spends a lot of time out in the sun and wind.

FACT BOX

• Most grown-ups can recognize at least 500 people from their faces. This includes family and friends, and also famous faces like stars of music, movies and sports.

• When you see your face in a mirror, it is not the face that other people see. It is reversed (swapped), left to right. This is why some people are surprised by the way they look in photographs.

• To see yourself as others see you, study a photograph of yourself. Compare it with your face in a mirror. Which one do you like best? Is it the most familiar one?

Disguise

If you want to disguise yourself, start with your face. This is the part that other people recognize most. You could wear a large hat and perhaps add or take off your glasses. A beard or a moustache might help, plus a scarf. The more of your face that you cover up, the less recognizable you become.

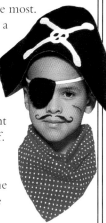

SKIN, HAIR AND NAILS

THE body is covered in skin – well, not quite. There are openings for parts such as the eyes, ears, nose and mouth. But the rest is skin. This body covering is flexible and stretchy, so you can move. It keeps body fluids and other substances inside. It keeps germs, dirt and other substances outside. Skin is always being worn away as you move around, get washed and dressed, grip and hold things, and rub against them. But skin is always growing just under the surface, to replace the parts that are worn away. Most of the skin over the body is covered with hair. Some of these hairs are thick and easily seen, like the hairs on your head. Other hairs are so small that you need a magnifying glass to see them. Only a few parts of the body are truly hairless, like the palms of the hands and soles of the feet.

Hair, like skin, keeps growing. Most people have about 100,000 hairs on their head. Each one grows for a couple years. It could reach more than 1 yard in length. Then it falls out and is replaced by a new hair.

With a magnifying glass, look very closely at the skin on different parts of the body. See how it varies. Some parts are smooth and flat. Others have lines and creases, especially around joints, where the skin stretches and bends a lot.

Handy skin
A hand has different kinds of skin – smooth, creased, thick, thin, hairless and hairy, as well as nails. Skin, hair and nails are all made from the substance called keratin. This is the same stuff that makes the claws, hooves and horns of other animals.

Close to skin
Under a powerful microscope, even the smoothest skin has tiny hills and valleys, lines and creases. Sweat oozes up through the tiny dotlike holes, called sweat pores.

Even closer to skin
The individual flakes of skin are microscopic dead cells, flattened and filled with tough keratin. They fall off the body by the thousand every minute.

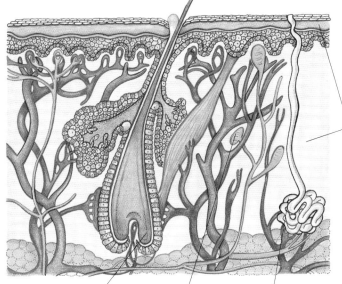

Epidermis

Dermis

Hair root   *Touch sensor*   *Sweat gland*

Giant hair

When you get this close to a hair, it does not look so smooth and shiny! The whole hair is dead, except for its very lowest part, the root, under the skin's surface.

Inside skin

Skin has two layers. The upper one is the epidermis. This keeps growing, to replace flakes of skin that are worn away. The lower layer is the dermis. It has tiny touch sensors, nerves and blood vessels.

Skin color

Different colors of skin and hair are due to different amounts of the very dark pigment (coloring substance) called melanin. Small patches of skin with slightly more melanin than surrounding skin are called freckles.

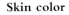

FACT BOX

• Spread out flat, the skin of a grown-up person would cover about 21 square feet, the same area as an office desk.

• The thickest skin is on the soles of the feet. In someone who does not wear shoes, it grows even thicker, for extra protection. It may be more than 1/4 inch thick.

• The thinnest skin is on the eyelids. It is less than two-hundredths of an inch thick.

• An average hair grows about four-hundredths of an inch every three days.

• An average fingernail grows about four-hundredths of an inch every seven days.

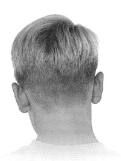 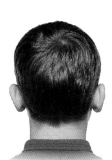 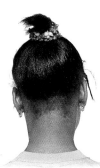

Hair types

Hair can be dark or light, thick (coarse) or thin (fine), and straight, wavy or curly. The length of the hair and the way it is styled greatly alter its appearance.

TOUCH AND FEELING

M A T E R I A L S

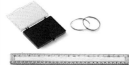

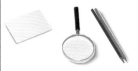

You will need: 2 pencils with sharp points, ruler, 2 rubber bands, ink pad, pale paper, magnifying glass.

WHEN you touch something, your skin tells you many things about it. You can feel whether it is hard or soft, hot or cold, rough or smooth, wet or dry. Touch comes from millions of microscopic sensors all over your skin. These detect light contact and heavy pressure, movement, temperature and other features. They send nerve signals to your brain, telling you what you are feeling. However, the touch sensors are not spread evenly all over the body. Some areas of skin have more of them, so they are more sensitive than other areas. Fingertips, with their swirly ridges, are very sensitive indeed to the slightest touch.

Sensitive points

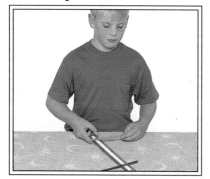

1 Fasten the pencils firmly to the ruler with the rubber band. Make one pencil point line up exactly with the 0 on the ruler scale.

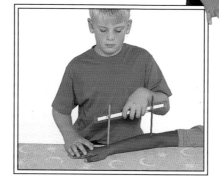

2 Ask a friend to close his eyes, or use a blindfold. Touch both pencil points gently at the same time on a patch of skin.

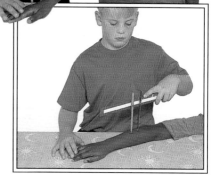

3 Does the friend feel two points, or one? Try again, reducing the gap between the pencils. The most sensitive skin detects the smallest gap.

Stamping fingerprints

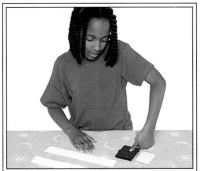

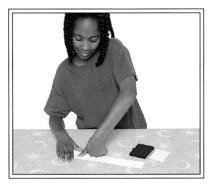

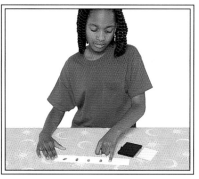

1 Swirly skin-ridge patterns on the fingers are called fingerprints. To see them, dab a finger or thumb on the ink pad with a rolling motion.

2 With the same rolling motion, dab the finger or thumb onto a strip of card. This transfers the ink and makes the print.

3 Make prints for all of your fingers and thumbs, and label them. Ask some friends to make their own sets of fingerprints, too.

Studying fingerprints

Study the sets of prints carefully under a magnifying glass. See how they have various patterns. These are called whorls (which are like part-spirals), arches and loops. With practice, can you recognize your own prints? Are the prints of your family members quite similar to your own?

Every print is different

No two people in the whole world have the same fingerprints. We all have different print patterns. This is why fingerprints can be used to prove that a person has been at a certain place. When the fingers touch a surface, they leave tiny traces of natural skin oil and sweat, in the same pattern as the prints. A special powder reveals the pattern.

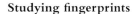

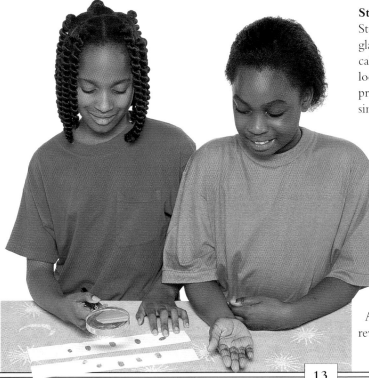

EYES AND SIGHT

THE body has five main senses that tell it about its surroundings. They are touch, sight, hearing, smell and taste. Seeing with the eyes is the most valuable sense. About half of the total knowledge and memory in the brain gets there through the eyes. This happens when you read words and look at pictures and diagrams, as you are doing now, and when you see people, objects and scenes around you. The eyes detect colors and patterns of light rays, turn these into nerve signals, and send them to the brain. Since vision is so important, everyone should have an eye test every year or two. (People who are blind or cannot see clearly rely on other senses more, like hearing and touch.)

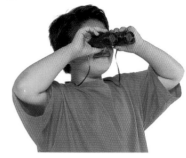

The eyes have their own small lenses, to focus light rays, for a clear view. Extra lenses like those in binoculars make things look larger and nearer.

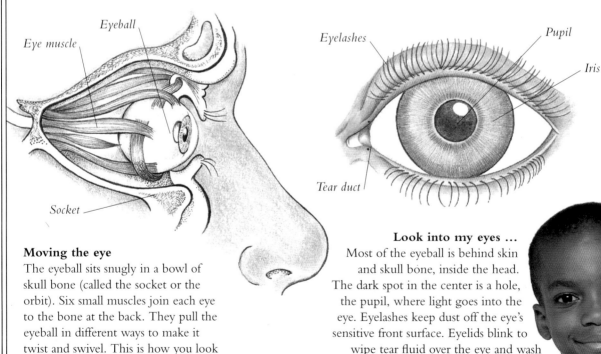

Moving the eye

The eyeball sits snugly in a bowl of skull bone (called the socket or the orbit). Six small muscles join each eye to the bone at the back. They pull the eyeball in different ways to make it twist and swivel. This is how you look up, down and to each side.

Look into my eyes …

Most of the eyeball is behind skin and skull bone, inside the head. The dark spot in the center is a hole, the pupil, where light goes into the eye. Eyelashes keep dust off the eye's sensitive front surface. Eyelids blink to wipe tear fluid over the eye and wash away dirt and germs.

Inside the eye

The cutaway view below shows the small and delicate parts inside the eyeball. Light comes in through the clear dome-shaped cornea at the front, and passes through the pupil, the circular hole in the iris. The light rays are focused (bent), so they shine a clear, sharp image onto the back of the eye. This is lined by the retina, which contains millions of light-sensitive cells. When the cells receive light rays, they create nerve signals which pass along the optic nerve to the brain.

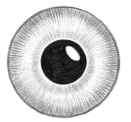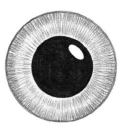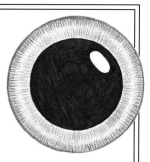

Iris and pupil

The eye's inside is very sensitive. Too much light is harmful. So the pupil gets small in bright light, to prevent damage. It widens in dim conditions, to see better in the dark. This happens by a change in size of the iris, the colored ring of muscle around the pupil.

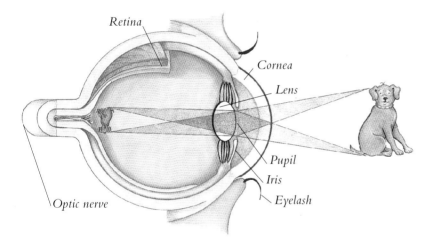

Retina

Cornea

Lens

Pupil

Iris

Eyelash

Optic nerve

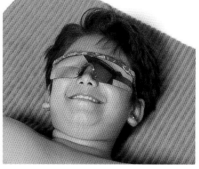

Eye care

Eyes can be harmed by dust, splashes of chemicals, objects like thrown stones or flies, and too much light – including bright sunshine. It is always wise to protect your eyes with goggles or sunglasses.

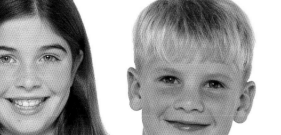

Eye color

Eye color is the color of the iris. It may be brown, green, blue, gray or nearly black. All new babies have blue eyes. The real color takes several months to develop.

TRICKING THE EYES

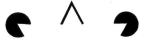

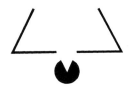

E YES cannot see everything, all around, all the time. When you look straight at something, to see its details, you miss what goes on around the sides. Also, we can make trick patterns and movements that the eye does not see in normal life. These fool the eye – rather, they fool the brain. It is your brain that analyzes the nerve signals from the eyes, identifies objects and colors and movements, and understands what you see.

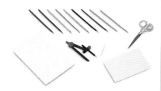

You will need: card, pair of compasses, pencils, scissors, toothpick.

This picture shows a white triangle – or does it? There seems to be a solid white triangle blocking out parts of the black disks and black triangle. The brain makes it up, as the most sensible reason for the pattern.

Optical illusions trick the brain. At one end, this looks like three round tubes. But at the other end, it looks like two square tubes. The pattern of lines on paper creates a puzzling picture which could not be a real object.

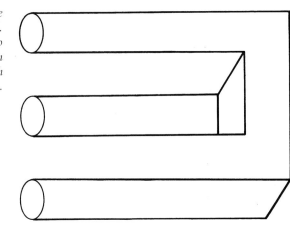

Hole-in-the-head?

If the brain cannot understand all of a scene, it makes up hidden parts and fills the gaps. Do that here, and the boy has an arrow through his head! But common sense tells us it is a trick. Sure enough, the arrow parts are joined by a curved piece of wire hidden in his hair.

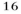

Spiral spinner

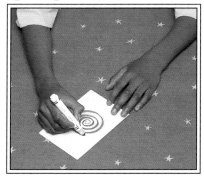

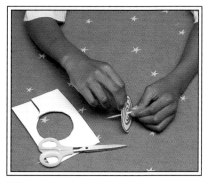

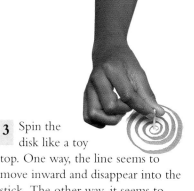

1 For the spiral spinner, draw a circle on the card, 6 inches across. Draw a spiral shape with the pencil first, to get the right shape. Then color it in.

2 Carefully cut the card around the circle's edge, to make a disk with the spiral on it. Push the toothpick through the disk's center, making sure the stick is a tight fit.

3 Spin the disk like a toy top. One way, the line seems to move inward and disappear into the stick. The other way, it seems to move out and fall off the disk's edge. Of course, it really goes nowhere!

Moving circles

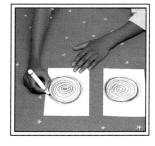

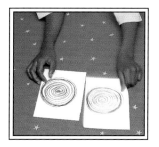

1 For moving circles, draw several sets of spirals or circles on a large white card. Make them clear and colorful. Do the same again, for a second set. Hold one card and move the other in small circles.

2 Can you make sense of what you see? Do the circles seem to rotate? This is a very unusual scene that the brain has trouble understanding. What effect do you see if you move both cards in small circles?

Color wheel

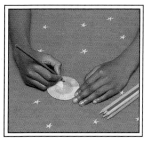

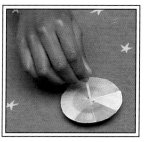

1 For a color wheel, divide a disk of card (4 inches across), into seven equal slices or segments (about 51° each). Color in the segments like a rainbow (the colors of the spectrum), in the correct order: red, orange, yellow, green, blue, indigo, violet.

2 Push a toothpick through the center, and spin fast. The colors merge into white (or perhaps gray). This is because white light is a mixture of many different colors of light: the spectrum. The spinning wheel merges these colors to form white.

EARS AND HEARING

Listen carefully. What can you hear? Even in the quietest place, there are sounds – whistling wind, rustling leaves, singing birds, a car or a plane. Hearing is the body sense that detects sound waves. These are invisible "ripples" that pass out from any object making a noise, whether it is a cat purrrrrrring or a hi-fi pounding out music. The ripples are vibrations, or fast back-and-forth movements, of the tiny floating molecules that make up air. Vibrations pass through air into your ears, which are inside the head, almost behind the eyes.

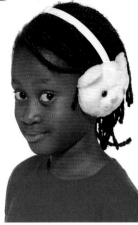

Protect your ears from extreme cold, or too-loud sounds, or very dusty air, with ear muffs. Like eyes, ears are delicate and easily harmed. Never push or poke anything into the ear canal. It should keep itself clean naturally.

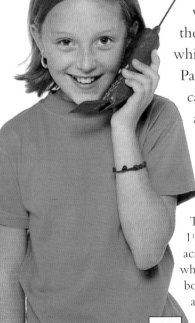

The inner parts of the ears detect the vibrations and change them into nerve signals, which go to the brain. Parts of the inner ears called semicircular canals also help to sense movements and gravity, to help you keep your balance.

Ear shapes
What we call "the ear" has little to do with hearing. It is simply a curved flap of skin and cartilage (gristle) on the side of the head. Ears come in many shapes and sizes, but this has little effect on hearing. They gather sound waves and funnel them into the ear canal.

On the phone
When you listen on the telephone, sound waves go from the earpiece, straight down the outer ear canal. This is the dark hole in the outer ear, and it is about $1\frac{1}{4}$ inches long. At its end is a thin piece of skin stretched across, called the eardrum (shown on the opposite page), which is about the size of your fingernail. The sound waves bounce off the eardrum and make it vibrate, or shake back and forth.

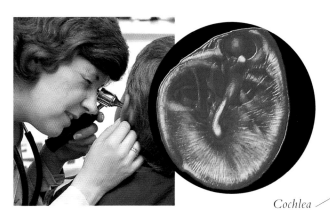

Semicircular canal   Anvil   Hammer

Cochlea

Stirrup

Eardrum   Ear canal

A doctor looks into the ear using an otoscope, to check for infections or other problems. The eardrum looks like a patch of thin reddish skin, with the hammer bone just behind it.

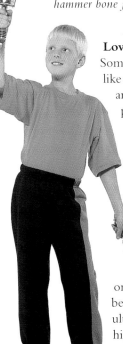

Low and high sounds

Some sounds are deep and booming, like thunder or a big drum. Others are high and shrill, such as a piercing scream or a cymbal. This is called pitch or frequency, and it is measured in Hertz (Hz). Human ears hear many frequencies, from the deepest notes at 25 Hz to extremely high ones at 15,000 Hz. In general, when big objects vibrate, they make deeper sounds. A large hand bell has a lower sound or musical note than a small hand bell. Some animals can hear ultrasounds. These are sounds too high-pitched for our ears to detect, like the squeaks of bats.

Inside the ear

Sound vibrations hit the eardrum and pass along three tiny bones, the hammer, anvil and stirrup, to fluid inside the snail-shaped cochlea. Here the vibrations are turned into nerve signals that go along the cochlear nerve to the brain.

Not too loud

The loudness of a sound is called its volume. It is measured in decibels. Sounds louder than about 85 to 90 decibels can damage the delicate inner parts of the ear, especially if they go on for a long time. So loud earphones or music speakers can harm your hearing. People who work near noisy machines, such as road drills and airplanes, wear earplugs to cut out the sound and protect their hearing.

LOUD AND QUIET

WHEN you hear a very loud noise, like a banging drum, do you turn away and put your hands over your ears? And when you try to hear something very quiet, like a whisper, do you lean forward and turn one ear toward it? Your body's position and movements help you to hear, and to keep your ears from being damaged by loud noises. These projects show how you can make sounds seem louder, and how you can see the vibrations of sound waves. The megaphone shown below is a funnel shape, like an extra-big mouth. It collects sound waves from your voice and makes them spread forward only. It also works the other way around, as an extra-big ear called an ear trumpet, which collects lots of sound waves.

Drums are fun but loud. The harder you hit them, the more the drum head (skin) vibrates, and the noisier it becomes. Bigger drums make lower, deeper bangs.

Whispers are quiet, and usually secret. If there are other sounds, like people talking or music playing, you may have to get very close to the whisperer.

Megaphone

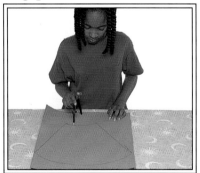

1 Carefully cut out this shape from a large sheet of thin cardboard. When rolled up and taped, it will form a funnel shape, which can be a megaphone or ear trumpet.

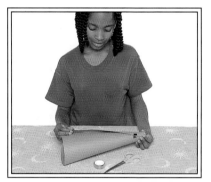

2 Roll the cardboard into a funnel or cone shape. Make the big end as wide as possible, and the small end about 1½ inches across. Tape the cardboard into this shape.

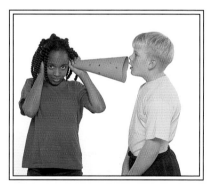

3 Listen normally to your friend talking, then with the funnel as an ear trumpet. Talk to the friend normally, then through the megaphone. Does it help?

Copy your ear

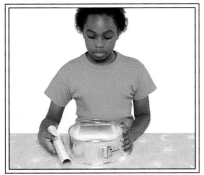

1 Cover one side of the pan with a sheet of plastic wrap. Make sure it is stretched tightly across, with no creases. If necessary, fasten it to the pan with tape.

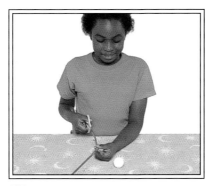

2 Push the short end of one straw into the long end of another. Carefully cut a few slits in the remaining long end so it splays out, ready for the ball.

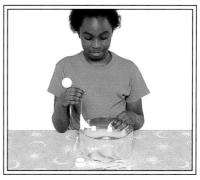

3 Tape the table-tennis ball onto the folded-back slits in the straw. Bend the straws at right angles and secure with tape. Tape the other straw to the plastic wrap as shown.

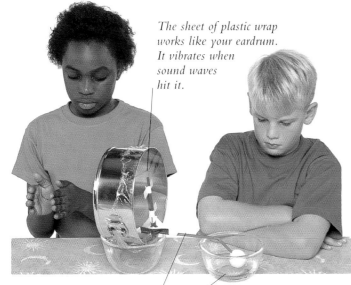

The sheet of plastic wrap works like your eardrum. It vibrates when sound waves hit it.

The straw works like your tiny ear bones. It passes vibrations along to the next part.

The bowl of water is like your cochlea. Vibrations spread as ripples across it.

MATERIALS

You will need: pan without base, like a baking pan, plastic wrap, tape, flexible plastic drinking straws, scissors, table-tennis ball, bowl or dish of water.

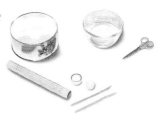

4 Support the baking pan on its side, on another bowl or on some books. Arrange and bend the straws so the table-tennis ball just touches the water in the bowl. This model setup is now like your ear! Make some sound waves near the pan, for example, by clapping. They hit the plastic wrap, which is like your eardrum. This vibrates and sends the vibrations along the straws, which work like the tiny ear bones. The ball makes ripples in the bowl, which is like the fluid-filled cochlea. As a result, you can see sound waves.

NOSE AND SMELL

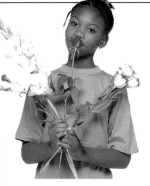

Enjoy the scents of the beautiful blooms. Sniff each type of flower in turn, and ask your friends which scent they like best. People have different personal preferences for scents and odors.

CAN you remember scents and smells for a long time? Perhaps you recall the smell of a holiday beach or the house of a relative. Smell is one of the body's five main senses. The smell area inside the nose detects tiny invisible particles, called odor molecules, floating in the air. Smell checks that our foods and drinks are not bad or rotten. It also warns us of danger, such as the nose-wrinkling smell of soft sinking mud, or the stench of stagnant, polluted water. Smell also gives pleasure, such as the lovely scents of flowers and perfumes and the aromas of good food.

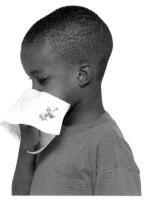

Your nose runs or gets blocked when you have an infection by germs, such as a cold. Get rid of the nasal mucus by sneezing or blowing into a tissue or a handkerchief.

Inside the nose
The nostrils are separated by a dividing wall, the septum. They lead into a large hole called the nasal cavity. When you breathe in, air comes through the nostrils, passes through the nasal cavity, and goes down the back, to the throat and windpipe. The smell area is in the top of the nasal cavity, and it is about the size of your thumbnail.

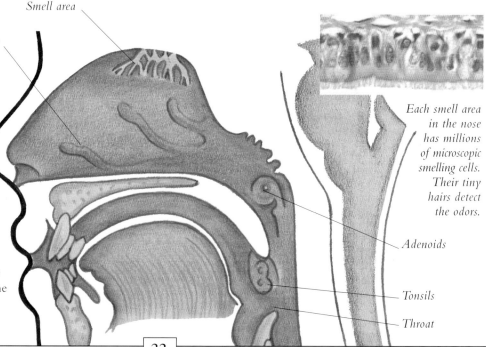

Smell area

Nasal cavity

Each smell area in the nose has millions of microscopic smelling cells. Their tiny hairs detect the odors.

Adenoids

Tonsils

Throat

A mouthwatering meal

Would you eat this well-cooked meal? Smell alone can make you hungry. Your brain recognizes food smells and gets your body ready. Watery saliva (spit) comes into your mouth, ready to moisten the chewing. This is why good foods smell "mouth-watering."

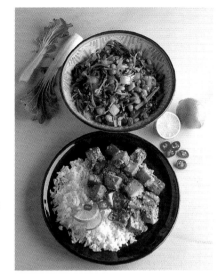

Bad and rotten!

Would you eat this old, rotting food? It looks awful, and if you could smell it, that would be even worse! If foods or drinks smell bad or rotten, they might cause food poisoning, so we avoid them. Smell gives us an early warning before we taste. This is a very important use of the sense of smell.

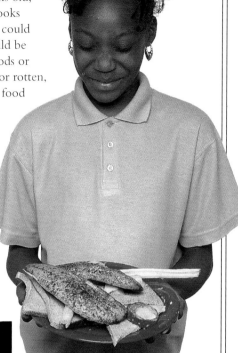

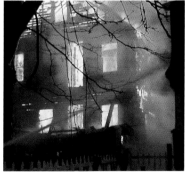

Overpowering fragrance

A few flowers are fine. But a whole field can be overpowering. Some smells are pleasant in normal amounts. But if they are too strong, they are not so nice. The amount or concentration of a smell alters its effects on us.

Sniff, sniff …

Is that smoke? This odor tells us at once about the risk of danger. The body becomes alert and ready for action. Animals react in the same way to the smell of a forest fire.

FACT BOX

• Most people could identify at least 10,000 different smells, if they had the time to try them all!

• A bloodhound can smell at least 1,000 times better than a person.

• The smell areas inside the top of the nose have 20 million smelling cells.

TONGUE AND TASTE

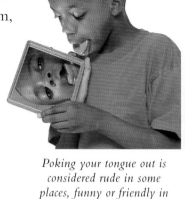

A S you eat your meal, you probably lick your lips slightly to clean them. This also moistens them, so they seal together well and stop food and drink dribbling out. Your tongue does many other jobs, too. It provides your sense of taste by detecting tiny particles called flavor molecules in foods and drinks. With smell, taste helps to tell you if foods are sour, rotten or bad, and should not be eaten. The tongue moves food around in your mouth, so you can chew it all properly. It also helps you to talk clearly, by moving around as you speak and make sounds.

Many animals use their tongues to clean their faces, whiskers, paws and other body parts. People do not need to, since we have hands, soap and water. But sometimes you might lick a stray bit of food or drink from your lips, or even your nose – if you can reach it!

Poking your tongue out is considered rude in some places, funny or friendly in others. Do it to yourself in a mirror. See the tongue's rough surface and the lumps (papillae).

Bumpy tongue

The top surface of the tongue is covered with small lumps and bumps, called papillae. There are different kinds, with larger ones at the back. All the papillae help to grip and rub food as you bite and chew.

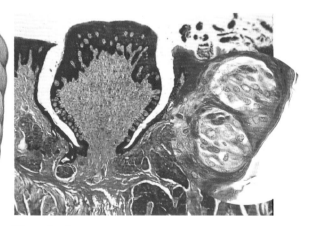

Taste buds

The microscope photograph, above left, shows a cut-through view of one papilla. Set into its lower edges (the stalk) are tiny taste buds. The enlarged view, above right, shows two taste buds with their tasting cells.

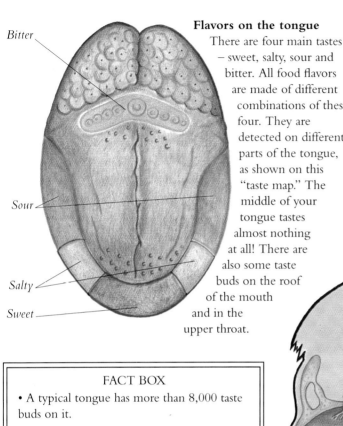

Bitter

Sour

Salty

Sweet

Flavors on the tongue

There are four main tastes – sweet, salty, sour and bitter. All food flavors are made of different combinations of these four. They are detected on different parts of the tongue, as shown on this "taste map." The middle of your tongue tastes almost nothing at all! There are also some taste buds on the roof of the mouth and in the upper throat.

Favorite flavors

Favorite tastes differ from one person to another. Most babies and young people like sweet foods. Some older people prefer salty, spicy or sour tastes. Hardness and texture are also important. Some foods seem slimy, slippery or lumpy. Which of the above foods do you like?

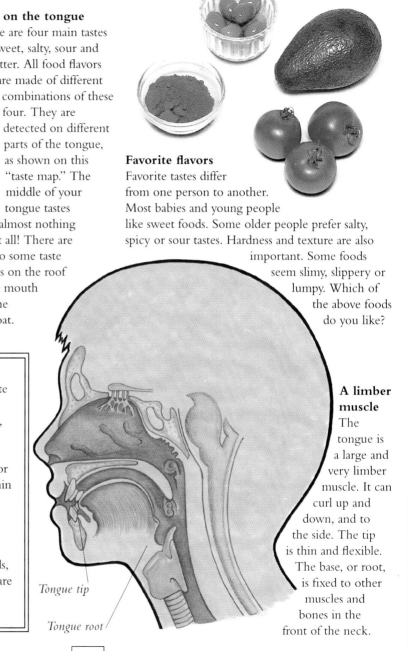

Tongue tip

Tongue root

A limber muscle

The tongue is a large and very limber muscle. It can curl up and down, and to the side. The tip is thin and flexible. The base, or root, is fixed to other muscles and bones in the front of the neck.

FACT BOX

• A typical tongue has more than 8,000 taste buds on it.

• Each taste bud has 20 to 30 "tasting cells" that detect flavors.

• The tasting cell in a taste bud lives only for 10 days, then it dies. But it is replaced within 12 hours by another one.

• Babies have more taste buds than adults, perhaps as many as 10,000.

• Older people usually have fewer taste buds, perhaps 5,000. So they may say that foods are bland and tasteless, while younger people with more taste buds disagree!

SMELL OR TASTE?

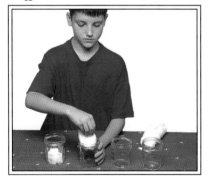

Some smells are similar. Sniff a spoonful of honey, then some jam. Can you tell the difference? They both smell sweet. Perhaps the jam has fruits in it, or the honey has real honeycomb.

WHEN you eat and drink, you use the senses of smell, taste, touch and sight – all together! You detect flavors using the taste buds on your tongue. You detect odors that float from the back of your mouth, up into the back of your nose, as you chew. You assess the temperature, hardness, moistness and texture of food by the different types of touch sensors in your mouth. This is different from taste. You also look at the food with your eyes to get an impression of how it might taste. All four of these senses tell you about the odors and flavors of foods and drinks. But what happens if some of these senses are blocked off? Is it harder to tell what you're eating?

M A T E R I A L S

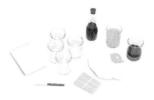

You will need: small pots or jars with lids, cotton, stick-on labels, pencil, notebook, drinks and juices such as apple, orange, grape, tomato, pineapple, coffee, milk and tea.

Sniff test

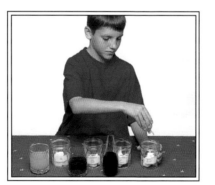

1 Try the sniff test on your friends. Put a lump of cotton into some small jars. Label each one. Make a list in your notebook of which juice or drink you will put into each jar. Keep the list secret!

2 Pour onto each lump of cotton the chosen drink or juice. Put on the lids. This stops the smells and odors escaping and mingling together in the air nearby, which could be confusing.

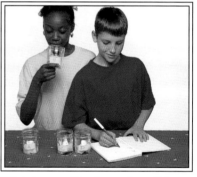

3 Ask your friends to take off the lids and sniff the jars, one by one, without looking inside. The only clue they have is smell. There is no sight, taste or touch. Can they identify what is in each jar?

Taste test

Fading tastes

Why do the first few lollipop licks taste best? If you keep eating the same thing, its taste gradually fades. The flavor molecules are still there, but the tongue becomes less sensitive to them. The same happens with smells. It is called habituation.

MATERIALS

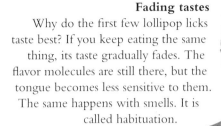

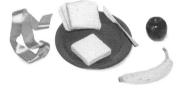

You will need: apple, banana, cheese, bread, pear, melon and similar pale and moist foods, safe knife, blindfold.

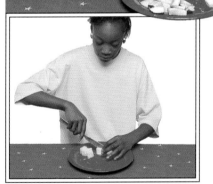

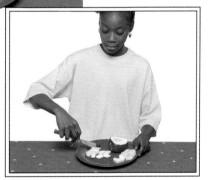

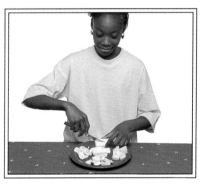

1 Try the taste test on your friends. Carefully peel each food and cut it into small cubes. Try to choose pale-looking foods, so there is little clue in the color. This helps to remove information gained by sight.

2 Cutting the food into cubes also helps to get rid of the clue of shape. This can be detected by sight and also by the touch sensors in the mouth. To make sure, ask the friend to put on a blindfold!

3 When you have cubed all the foods, ask your friend to chew each one a few times, then swallow it. There are hardly any clues from smell or touch. Are the foods easy to identify by taste alone?

NERVES AND BRAIN

HAVE you used your brain today? Perhaps you have thought hard to solve a problem, or managed to remember something difficult. Thoughts, memories, ideas and wishes all happen in the brain. They are in the form of tiny electrical pulses, called nerve signals. These whiz about among the brain's complicated network of long, thin nerves – millions of them. Much more happens in the brain, too. It is where you feel emotions like love, fear and anger. It is where signals come to, from the senses. It is where you decide to make movements and actions. It is also the control center for all your body's inner processes, like heartbeat, breathing and digesting food. The brain is truly the control center for the whole body.

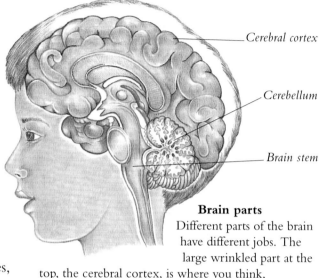

Cerebral cortex

Cerebellum

Brain stem

Brain parts
Different parts of the brain have different jobs. The large wrinkled part at the top, the cerebral cortex, is where you think, remember, decide and become aware of what is happening. The cerebellum at the lower rear makes your movements smooth and coordinated. The lowest part, the brain stem, controls basic life processes like heartbeat.

Safe brain
The brain is very delicate. But it is well protected against knocks by the hard skull bone around it. Even so, it is always wise to wear a safety hat or helmet for extra protection, in case you get a bump on the head.

Seeing the brain
Medical scanners used in hospitals can see inside the head, without any pain or damage (and without cutting it open)! They reveal any injury or disease. This false-color picture shows the wrinkled cerebral cortex and the two eyes with their optic nerves.

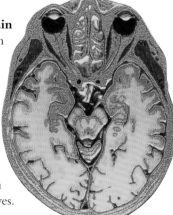

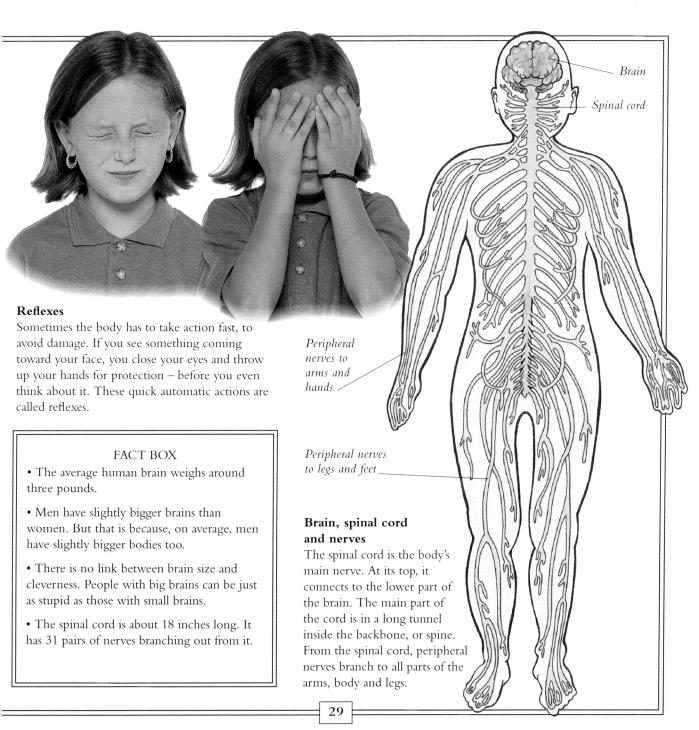

Brain

Spinal cord

Reflexes

Sometimes the body has to take action fast, to avoid damage. If you see something coming toward your face, you close your eyes and throw up your hands for protection – before you even think about it. These quick automatic actions are called reflexes.

Peripheral nerves to arms and hands

Peripheral nerves to legs and feet

FACT BOX

• The average human brain weighs around three pounds.

• Men have slightly bigger brains than women. But that is because, on average, men have slightly bigger bodies too.

• There is no link between brain size and cleverness. People with big brains can be just as stupid as those with small brains.

• The spinal cord is about 18 inches long. It has 31 pairs of nerves branching out from it.

Brain, spinal cord and nerves

The spinal cord is the body's main nerve. At its top, it connects to the lower part of the brain. The main part of the cord is in a long tunnel inside the backbone, or spine. From the spinal cord, peripheral nerves branch to all parts of the arms, body and legs.

AWAKE AND ASLEEP

WHEN you wake up in the morning, and it feels as if you have had a good rest, most of your body has. But some parts, like your heart and lungs, have been working all night. So has your brain. During sleep, it is busy doing various activities. No one knows exactly what, or why. But they must be important, because people who cannot sleep become confused, and suffer headaches and pains. They may even collapse.

When the brain and body need sleep, they tell you by feeling tired. If you ignore this, they go to sleep anyway. Young children can drop off almost anywhere!

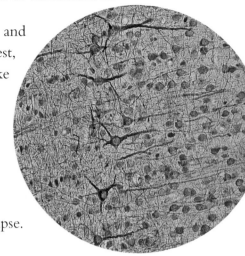

Nerve cells
Like other parts of the body, the brain and nerves are made of cells. They are called nerve cells or neurons. They have long, thin branches that connect to other nerve cells. There are about 100 billion nerve cells in the brain, forming an immense network of pathways for nerve signals.

Brain centers
Different parts of the brain's outer surface, the cerebral cortex, deal with nerve signals coming from the senses. The signals from the eyes arrive at the seeing (visual) center, at the back. They are sorted and compared with patterns of signals already in the brain's memory. In this way, you recognize what you see. Other senses have similar centers.

Movement planning center

Movement center

Touch center

Taste center

Other sight centers

Main sight center

Talking center

Hearing center

Smell center (in middle of brain)

Cerebellum for movement coordination

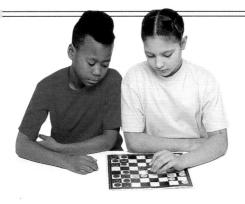

The sides of the brain

The brain looks the same on each side. But the sides have different main activities. The left side takes charge in logic and reasoning, like solving problems in a step-by-step way, working with numbers, writing and speaking words. The right side tends to take the lead in creative and artistic processes like having ideas, recognizing patterns, painting pictures and making music.

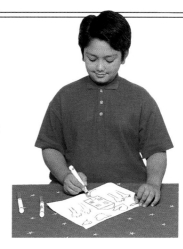

Falling asleep   *REM (dreaming) sleep*   *Waking up*

Deep sleep   *One hour*

Sleep and dreams

When you nod off each night, first you go into deep sleep. Body processes such as heartbeat and breathing slow down, and muscles relax. But after a time, these speed up slightly. Muscles twitch and eyes flick about under closed lids. This is REM (rapid eye movement) sleep, when dreams usually happen. Then you go into deep sleep again, and so on, through the night.

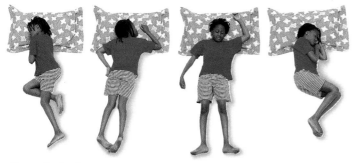

Busy in bed

You do not stay completely still all night. Otherwise you would squash the nerves, blood vessels and other body parts you are lying on. You move and shift your position as many as 50 times.

FACT BOX
- A newborn baby needs about 20 hours of sleep each day.

- A 10-year-old needs about 10 hours' sleep each night.

- An adult needs seven to eight hours' sleep each night.

- But these are all averages. Some people have less sleep, others more. But whatever your sleep needs are, don't fight them.

MEMORIES

THERE is not one place in the brain for memories. They seem to be spread through several brain parts. Memories are probably complicated connections and pathways for nerve signals among the brain's millions of nerve cells. There are two stages to making a memory. One is to remember, which is to store the information in your brain. The other is to recall it, which is to find it again. You can play a sport or musical instrument better with practice – and you can do the same with memories. The more you try and learn to remember, the better you should become. There are also a few memory aids, short-cuts and "tricks" that you can use, as shown here.

M A T E R I A L S

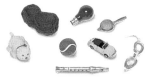

You will need for the memory tray: a selection of household toys, ornaments, utensils and similar small items.

Some people write about their lives in a diary. This is a memory aid. They can look up a day which happened long ago. From a few words in the diary, they can begin to recall many other things that happened. The few words act as a memory trigger.

Memory test

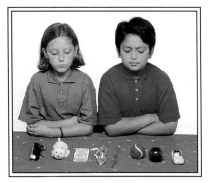

1 Lay out a row of about eight or ten small and everyday objects on a table. A friend looks at them for about 20 seconds. He or she tries to remember their names and their positions in the row.

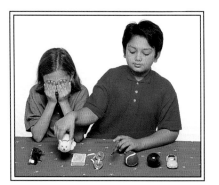

2 The friend closes eyes, and you move two objects, to swap their positions. The friend then looks again, and tries to identify the moved items. This is usually easier than remembering all the items in order.

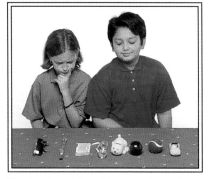

3 Study all the objects again and try to memorize them. One trick is to make a word from the first letter of each of their names. Or try to include their names in a silly story, which makes them easier to recall.

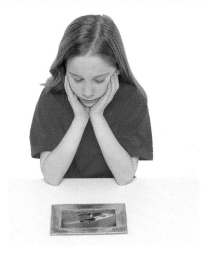

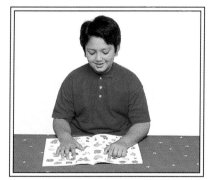

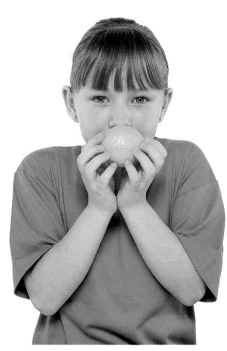

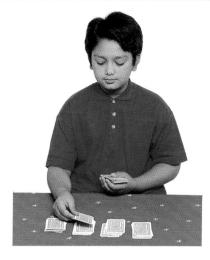

Memories in smells and pictures

A picture or a smell triggers your memory by taking your mind back to where and when you saw what is in the picture or smelled the smell.

Luck and judgment

Some games are partly luck. But you can usually play them better if you train yourself to remember certain things. You can work out where a card is in the deck by remembering the cards before it.

Picture memory game

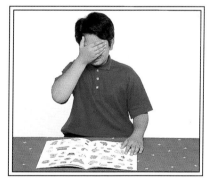

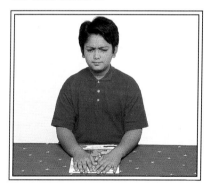

1 Some people find that they can remember pictures better than numbers and words. Try this picture memory test. Look at pictures in a book for 20 seconds. Note their shapes, colors and other details.

2 Now concentrate on the picture memories in your mind. Keep going through each part, so it stays "fresh." Repeat the details of the shapes, shading and colors, and the names of any objects.

3 After another 20 seconds, close the book and describe the pictures or draw them. Get friends to try the same test. Do it several times. With practice, you should gradually become more skilled.

FOOD FOR THE BODY

IF you do not eat a meal for a few hours, you soon begin to feel hungry. This is your body's way of telling you that it needs more energy, to power its thousands of chemical life processes. And it needs more nutrients (raw materials) too, for running repairs, growth and body maintenance. So you eat. Food contains both energy and nutrients. Some animals eat only one kind of food. Pandas feed on bamboo, and koalas munch solely on eucalyptus leaves. But the human body needs a wide variety of foods to stay healthy. In particular, fresh vegetables and fruits are very good for the body.

Imagine what you eat in a typical month. It probably adds up to about 100 pounds in weight of food, plus 50 quarts of drinks. Even more amazing, it turns into you!

Carbohydrates and fiber
Carbohydrates are the body's main energy source. They are found in rice, potatoes, bread and pasta. Fiber (roughage) is not fully digested but it gives food bulk and texture, and it keeps the intestines working. Whole grains (oats, for example), vegetables and fruit have plenty of fiber.

Protein and fat
Proteins provide raw materials for maintenance and growth. Proteins are found in meat, fish, dairy produce, and some vegetables such as peas and beans. Fats are needed in fairly small amounts for healthy nerves and other body parts.

Food gives you energy

The energy in foods is measured in calories. A slice of whole-meal bread contains about 60 calories, plus useful vitamins, minerals and fiber. A bar of chocolate contains 250 calories but little else. Your energy needs depend mainly on how active you are. If you eat too much high-energy food, such as cookies or chips, the body converts the extra calories to fat.

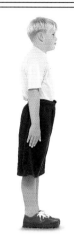

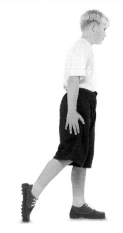

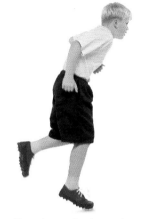

Resting uses about 1 calorie per minute.

Walking or gentle activity uses 3 calories per minute.

Running or hard exercise uses 7 calories per minute.

Fruit

Most fruits, such as passion fruit and strawberries, are a good source of sugar, for energy, as well as vitamins, minerals and fiber.

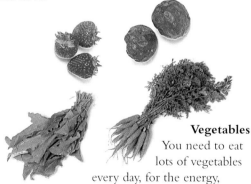

Vegetables

You need to eat lots of vegetables every day, for the energy, fiber, vitamins and minerals they provide. Dark green vegetables are especially good for you.

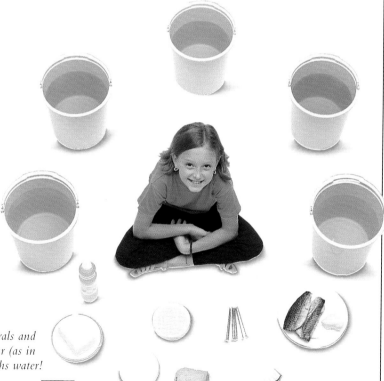

The body contains an amazing assortment of minerals and substances, including iron (as in nails) and sulphur (as in match-heads). And the body is three-fifths water!

35

MOUTH AND TEETH

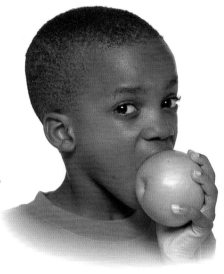

THE first stop for the body's food is its mouth, with its various parts: lips, teeth, tongue and cheeks. Each part has a job to do. The teeth bite off pieces of food, and chew and squash and mash them. The lips open to let the food in, then seal together so that it does not fall out. The cheeks bulge as the tongue moves the food around between the teeth, for thorough chewing. As food is chewed, it is mixed with watery saliva, or spit, to make it soft and moist. Then the tongue pushes the mashed lump of food back into the throat, for swallowing down into the stomach. All the mouth's chewing work helps digest food.

If an item of food is too big for your mouth, you can try to break it with your fingers, or cut it up with a knife. But the easiest way is usually to bite off a piece, using your sharp front teeth, the incisors.

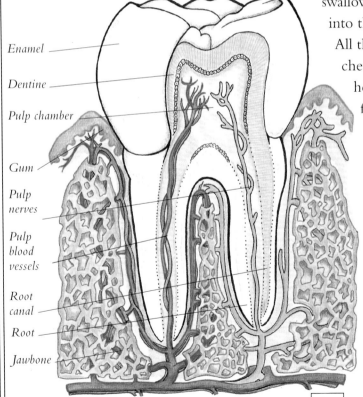

Enamel

Dentine

Pulp chamber

Gum

Pulp nerves

Pulp blood vessels

Root canal

Root

Jawbone

Inside a tooth

A tooth's upper part, the crown, is covered by whitish enamel, the hardest substance in the body. Underneath is dentine, slightly softer to absorb knocks and great pressure. The tooth's lower part, the root, anchors it in the jawbone. At the center is a living pulp of blood vessels to provide nourishment, and nerves that warn of too much pressure, or dental decay – toothache! Clean your teeth morning and night, after every meal if possible, to remove the leftover food and germs that cause tooth decay. Visit the dentist regularly for a check on teeth and gums, and for advice on cleaning and flossing teeth.

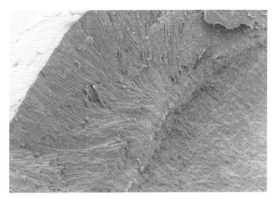

Enamel
This cross-section of a tooth, magnified 275 times, shows that tooth enamel is formed from thousands of tiny rods.

Diets of the dead
We can tell what people have eaten, even after they die, from the shapes of their teeth, and the tiny marks and scratches on the tooth surface. These clues show that prehistoric people such as Heidelberg Man, who lived perhaps a half million years ago, ate plenty of tough plant roots and shoots.

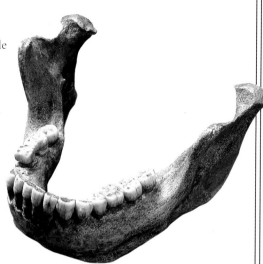

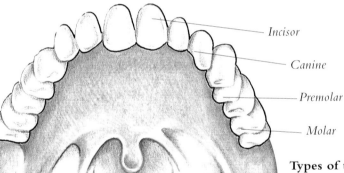

Incisor

Canine

Premolar

Molar

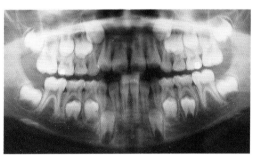

Types of teeth
The four main kinds of teeth are shaped to do different jobs. Incisors at the front are wide and sharp-edged like chisels, for biting and nibbling. Canines are longer and more pointed, to tear and rip. Premolars and molars at the back are broad and fairly flat, to squash and crush.

Hidden teeth
A dental X-ray shows a child's adult teeth under its milk teeth. From about the age of six, the milk teeth fall out and are replaced by the adult or permanent teeth. In each half of each jaw (upper and lower) a child has two incisors, one canine and two molars, making a total of 20 teeth. An adult has two incisors, one canine, two premolars and three molars, making a total of 32 teeth.

THE DIGESTIVE SYSTEM

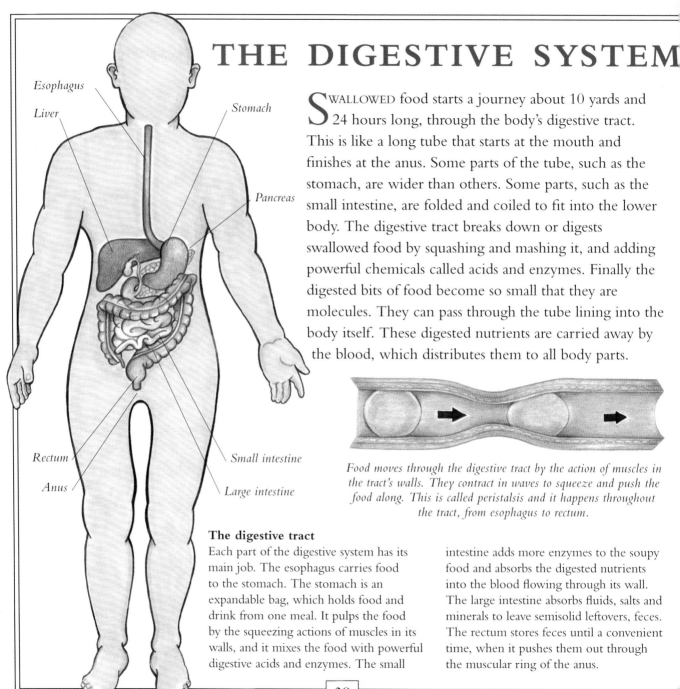

Esophagus
Liver
Stomach
Pancreas
Rectum
Anus
Small intestine
Large intestine

SWALLOWED food starts a journey about 10 yards and 24 hours long, through the body's digestive tract. This is like a long tube that starts at the mouth and finishes at the anus. Some parts of the tube, such as the stomach, are wider than others. Some parts, such as the small intestine, are folded and coiled to fit into the lower body. The digestive tract breaks down or digests swallowed food by squashing and mashing it, and adding powerful chemicals called acids and enzymes. Finally the digested bits of food become so small that they are molecules. They can pass through the tube lining into the body itself. These digested nutrients are carried away by the blood, which distributes them to all body parts.

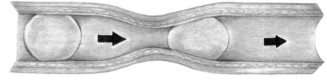

Food moves through the digestive tract by the action of muscles in the tract's walls. They contract in waves to squeeze and push the food along. This is called peristalsis and it happens throughout the tract, from esophagus to rectum.

The digestive tract

Each part of the digestive system has its main job. The esophagus carries food to the stomach. The stomach is an expandable bag, which holds food and drink from one meal. It pulps the food by the squeezing actions of muscles in its walls, and it mixes the food with powerful digestive acids and enzymes. The small intestine adds more enzymes to the soupy food and absorbs the digested nutrients into the blood flowing through its wall. The large intestine absorbs fluids, salts and minerals to leave semisolid leftovers, feces. The rectum stores feces until a convenient time, when it pushes them out through the muscular ring of the anus.

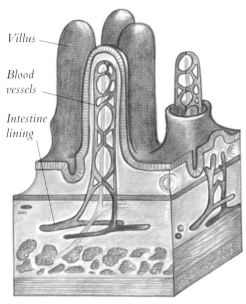

Villus

Blood
vessels

Intestine
lining

Digestion times

The amount of time it takes for food to travel through your digestive system varies, depending on how easy it is to digest.

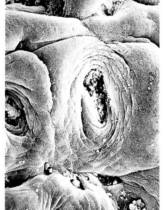

Mouth
(minutes for
each swallow)

Esophagus
(seconds for each
swallow)

Stomach
(hours 1 to 6)

Small intestine
(hours 2 to 15)

Large intestine
(hours 6 to 24)

Anus
(hours 12 to 24)

Inside the intestine

The small intestine lining has thousands of tiny short hairlike parts called villi. These give a large surface area for absorbing food. Each villus has blood vessels that carry the digested food away to where it is needed.

Digestive juices

Tiny pits in the lining of the stomach (*above*) and between the villi of the small intestine ooze digestive juices. These consist of enzymes and powerful acids, which break down the food.

FACT BOX

• The esophagus is about 10 inches long and 1 inch wide. Its walls are very muscular.

• The stomach can expand to hold more than $1\frac{1}{2}$ quarts of foods and fluids.

• The small intestine is 20 feet long and 1 inch wide.

• The large intestine, or colon, is 5 feet long and about 2 inches wide.

• The rectum is 6 inches long and about 2 inches wide.

Parts of the system

The liver and pancreas are not part of the digestive tract, but they are part of the digestive system. The liver receives blood from the small intestine, loaded with nutrients. It processes, stores, alters and distributes them according to the body's needs. The pancreas makes digestive enzymes that pour into the small intestine, to help food breakdown.

EATING AND DRINKING

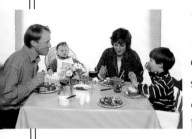

Many important events include food, from the ice cream and cake of a birthday party to the many courses of a huge banquet for kings or presidents.

FOOD provides fuel for the body, and much more. It gives us great enjoyment and pleasure, as we eat a delicious meal. For some people, cooking food is a skilled job or an interesting pastime – or even an obsession! Food also gives us the opportunity to take a break and meet others. When we sit down for a meal, we have time to pause from the rush of the day, think and consider what to do next. We can appreciate the meal and drinks, and chat and talk with family and friends. Trying to eat while moving about or doing other things can cause problems. We may not chew thoroughly, and rushed food may even choke us.

M A T E R I A L S

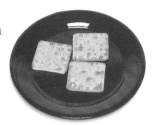

You will need: crackers or dry cookies (plus something to drink).

Make your mouth water

A moist mouth
Watery saliva, or spit, is made in three pairs of salivary glands around the face. Saliva softens and moistens food as you chew, so that you can mash it to a squishy pulp and swallow it easily. It also begins the chemical breakdown (digestion) of the starch in food. Normally we do not notice saliva and what it does, since many foods are moist. But if you eat very-dry foods, you soon notice its absence.

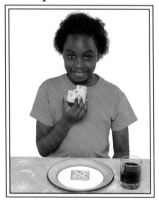

1 Bite off and chew a piece of cracker. Chew slowly. Can you feel the saliva making the dry cracker damp and soft? Swallow, and eat another piece.

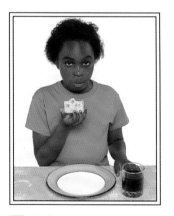

2 And eat some more. The salivary glands make about 1 quart of saliva daily. But there is only a limited amount in a few minutes, less than 4 ounces.

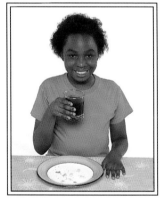

3 How many crackers can you eat, before they become too dry and hard to chew? Your saliva is used up, and you need a drink to finish the job.

Strange-looking foods

Before we eat, we check that a meal is safe to eat. We sniff for its smell, and we look at it to identify the foods. Are they the right shape and color? If these appear odd, such as different colors from normal, we might be worried about eating them. This is a natural reaction or instinct. Blue foods, such as this blue pasta, look especially odd. Can you think of more than two or three natural, safe blue foods?

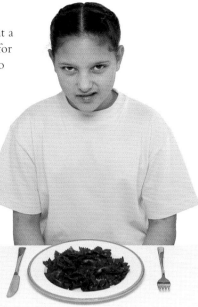

Funny texture

The appearance of food in terms of texture is important too. Fish sticks, fried eggs and vegetables normally look tasty, but if you mash them up, you probably wouldn't want them anymore!

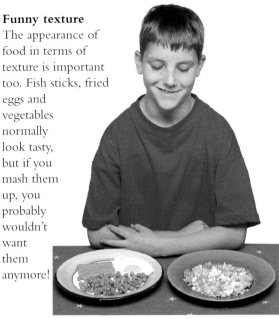

MATERIALS

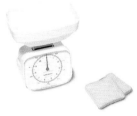

You will need: selection of foods, such as bread, scales, supervised use of an oven.

The body needs about 3 quarts of water every day. Some of this comes in as foods, the rest as drinks. How much of a food is water?

Water in food

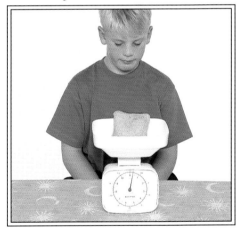

1 Carefully weigh the chosen piece of food, such as a slice of bread. Ask an adult to put the food in a suitable container in the oven, next time it is on.

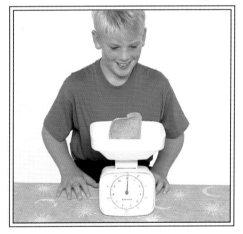

2 Heat the food until it is dry, but not burned. Let the food cool. Remove the food and weigh it again. What proportion was water, now evaporated?

BODY WASTES

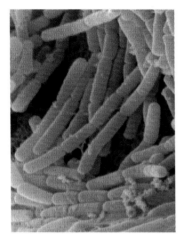

Not all microbes are harmful germs. These friendly bacteria live in everyone's intestines, and they help with digestion.

Aᴌᴌ animals produce waste, from small mouse droppings to huge mounds of elephant dung. The human body does, too. Like cats, dogs and similar creatures, it makes two main kinds of wastes. There are solid wastes, also called feces or bowel movements (and many other names!), and liquid wastes, also known as urine or "water" (and many other names!). These two kinds of wastes have very different origins. Feces are the leftovers at the end of the digestive process. They come out of the end of the digestive tract. Urine is mainly chemical waste and excess water filtered from the blood by the parts called the kidneys. It comes from the bladder. The body also produces a waste gas called carbon dioxide, which it breathes out through the lungs.

Listen to your tummy

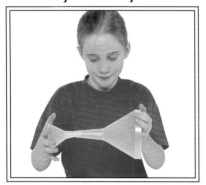

1 You can hear wastes gurgling through the guts, with two funnels. Push the spouts of the two funnels together tightly.

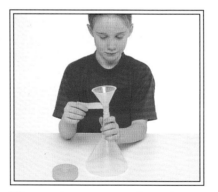

2 Tape the spouts together. The large funnel acts as a sound-collector for body noises such as digestion or heartbeat.

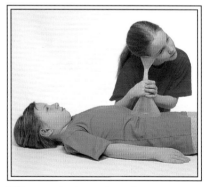

3 Press the large funnel onto a friend's abdomen, and the small one around your ear. Can you hear food slurping and gases bubbling?

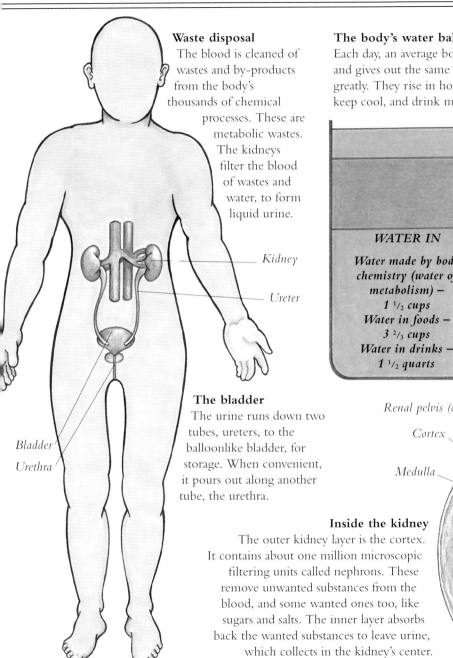

Waste disposal

The blood is cleaned of wastes and by-products from the body's thousands of chemical processes. These are metabolic wastes. The kidneys filter the blood of wastes and water, to form liquid urine.

Kidney

Ureter

Bladder

Urethra

The bladder

The urine runs down two tubes, ureters, to the balloonlike bladder, for storage. When convenient, it pours out along another tube, the urethra.

The body's water balance

Each day, an average body takes in about 3 quarts of water, and gives out the same amount. But these quantities vary greatly. They rise in hot weather, as you sweat more to keep cool, and drink more to replace this perspired water.

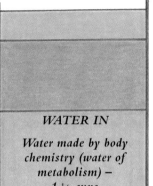

WATER IN

Water made by body chemistry (water of metabolism) –
1 ¹/₂ cups
Water in foods –
3 ²/₃ cups
Water in drinks –
1 ¹/₂ quarts

WATER OUT

Water in feces –
¹/₂ cup
Water in urine –
1 ¹/₂ quarts
Water in sweat and as vapor in breathed-out air –
3 ³/₄ cups

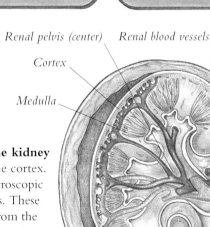

Renal pelvis (center)   *Renal blood vessels*

Cortex

Medulla

Ureter

Inside the kidney

The outer kidney layer is the cortex. It contains about one million microscopic filtering units called nephrons. These remove unwanted substances from the blood, and some wanted ones too, like sugars and salts. The inner layer absorbs back the wanted substances to leave urine, which collects in the kidney's center.

LUNGS AND BREATHING

ALL animals and plants need oxygen for life. Oxygen is an invisible gas in the air around us. It is required for part of the chemical changes that happen in every body cell, to break down digested foods and nutrients, and get the energy from them. This energy powers muscles and the body's life processes. The series of chemical changes is called aerobic respiration. The body cannot store oxygen, so it must get fresh supplies every minute. It does this by breathing (respiring). The parts involved in breathing and absorbing oxygen from the air are called the respiratory system. They include the nose, throat, windpipe (trachea) and the two spongy, cone-shaped lungs in the chest.

The two lungs normally hold about 13 cubic feet of air. But when the body is very active, it needs more oxygen. If you breathe in very deeply, the lungs hold over 25 cubic feet of air.

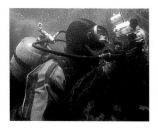

Well-trained humans can hold their breath for a minute or so when swimming underwater. But for longer periods, we need to take our own oxygen supply to breathe. This is contained as pressurized air or oxygen inside scuba tanks.

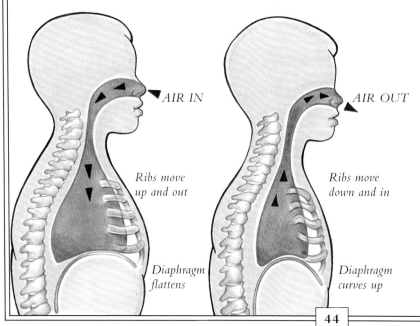

AIR IN

Ribs move up and out

Diaphragm flattens

AIR OUT

Ribs move down and in

Diaphragm curves up

Muscles for breathing

The movements of breathing are called bodily respiration. They are made by two main sets of muscles. One is the diaphragm, a sheet of muscle under the lungs. The other set is the intercostals, short muscles between each pair of ribs.

In and out

To breathe in, the diaphragm contracts to become shorter and flatter, and the lungs stretch downward. The intercostals contract, pulling up the ribs, which stretches the lungs forward. The stretched lungs suck in air. To breathe out, the diaphragm and intercostals relax. The stretched lungs spring back, and blow out air.

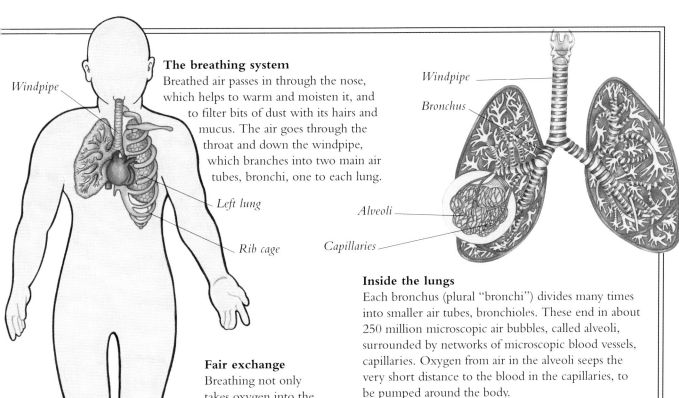

The breathing system

Breathed air passes in through the nose, which helps to warm and moisten it, and to filter bits of dust with its hairs and mucus. The air goes through the throat and down the windpipe, which branches into two main air tubes, bronchi, one to each lung.

Windpipe

Left lung

Rib cage

Windpipe

Bronchus

Alveoli

Capillaries

Inside the lungs

Each bronchus (plural "bronchi") divides many times into smaller air tubes, bronchioles. These end in about 250 million microscopic air bubbles, called alveoli, surrounded by networks of microscopic blood vessels, capillaries. Oxygen from air in the alveoli seeps the very short distance to the blood in the capillaries, to be pumped around the body.

Fair exchange

Breathing not only takes oxygen into the body. It also gets rid of carbon dioxide, a waste product made in cells by aerobic respiration. This is collected by the blood and passes into the air in the lungs, for breathing out. If carbon dioxide built up in the blood, it would soon poison the body.

FACT BOX

• At rest, an average person breathes in and out about 14 to 16 times per minute.

• After lots of exercise, this can rise to more than 60 times per minute.

• At rest, an average person breathes in and out about 30 cubic inches of air.

• After lots of exercise, this can rise to more than 10 cubic feet of air with each breath.

• At rest, new babies breathe 40 to 50 times each minute, much faster than adults. This slows to 25 times per minute by the age of 5 years.

BREATHED-IN AIR
Nitrogen – 78 percent
Oxygen – 21 percent
Carbon dioxide – 0.04 percent
Plus other gases

BREATHED-OUT AIR
Nitrogen – 79 percent
Oxygen – 16 percent
Carbon dioxide – 4 percent
Plus other gases

BREATHING AND BLOWING

Breathing has many uses, in addition to obtaining oxygen. As the moving air passes through your voice-box or larynx in your neck, it allows you to talk and sing. If you purse your lips or blow through a narrow gap between your fingers, you can whistle. If you blow out hard, you can spin toy windmills and inflate balloons. When you blow out forcefully like this, you use extra muscles in your abdomen and chest. Breathing also works many musical instruments, from recorders to trumpets and tubas.

Hold a toy windmill in front of your mouth and breathe normally. Does it spin? Blow gently, then hard. Does it move? Try different breathing-type actions such as talking, shouting and whistling. Which spins the windmill fastest?

Don't blow too hard

As you blow up a balloon, you force air from your lungs up your windpipe and mouth, into the balloon. But this requires lots of muscle power in your chest and abdomen and great air pressure in your lungs. If you try too hard for too long, it could damage the lungs' delicate air bubbles (alveoli) that take in oxygen. A proper air pump for blowing up balloons is much less risky!

How fast do you breathe?

Find out using a stopwatch or similar timepiece, to time your breaths. Breathing in, then out, is one breath. Count the number of breaths in 30 seconds and double it to find the rate per minute. Try various activities and see how they affect your breathing rate.

Sit at rest for 5 minutes and count your breaths. How do you compare with the average rates on the previous page? Next, say your favorite nursery rhyme several times, and count your breathing rate as you do this. (Talking as you breathe out is the out-breath.) Then run on the spot for 5 minutes, and count the rate again. How fast does it get?

MATERIALS

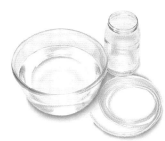

You will need: water, large shallow bowl, large glass or clear plastic see-through jar or jug, length of tubing or garden hose or similar flexible pipe.

The breath machine
You can compare the amounts of air you breathe when doing different actions, using this homemade version of the scientific device called a spirometer. You breathe out air through the tube, and it bubbles into the water-filled jar and pushes the water out. The lower the water level in the jar after the breath, the bigger the volume of that breath.

Water level in jar shows volume of breathed-out air.

4 After breathing in from the air, breathe out carefully into the tube.

Warning
Never breathe in through the tube, or you could cough and choke on water!

How much air?

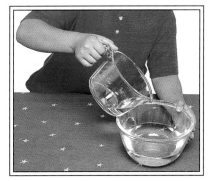

1 Half-fill the large shallow bowl with water and put it on a firm surface. Also, completely fill the large jar with water.

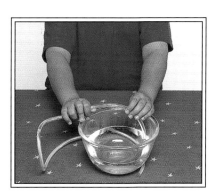

2 Place the tube into the water, ready to place the jar on top. With your hand sealed over the jar's mouth, quickly turn it upside down.

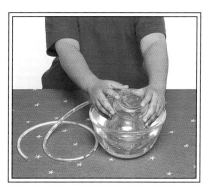

3 Put the jar in the bowl, take your hand away and the water should stay in the jar. Put one end of the tube under the rim, into the jar.

TALKING

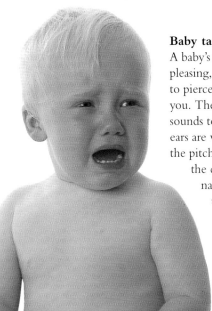

H AVE you been told off for talking too much? Who hasn't? Too much chat is sometimes out of place. But speech is a natural, everyday part of life. Humans are generally social creatures and like to be in groups with family and friends. Speech is our main form of communication. We talk about foods and drinks, sports and the weather, wishes and wants, and how we think and feel. The sounds of speech are made possible by the vocal cords in the larynx (voice box), which is in the neck. This is part of the respiratory system (the lungs and the windpipe). We also communicate by making facial expressions such as smiles and frowns, by using our hands, and by our general body posture, behavior and movements. This is called body language. In the right situation, a small yet silent movement of part of the body can say more than words ever could.

Birds such as parrots and mynahs can imitate many sounds, from the noise of a car or telephone to words of human speech. But the bird does not understand or mean what it says.

Baby talk
A baby's gurgle is very pleasing, but its cry seems to pierce right through you. These are difficult sounds to ignore. Human ears are very sensitive to the pitch or frequency of the cry, and we naturally want to try and stop it by helping the baby. This is part of nature. Other animals do the same for their offspring.

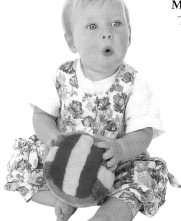

Meaning without talking
The vocal cords make many other vocal sounds, besides speech. We laugh, cry, sob and hum. These and many other sounds made by the cords are called vocalizations. They also convey messages such as happiness or sadness. The loudness and other features of the sound are also important. A loud, short shout usually means a warning or attracts attention. Whispering sweet nothings shows affection!

Spiral spinner

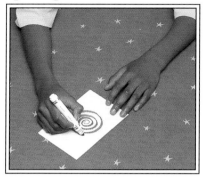

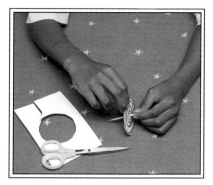

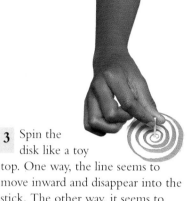

1 For the spiral spinner, draw a circle on the card, 6 inches across. Draw a spiral shape with the pencil first, to get the right shape. Then color it in.

2 Carefully cut the card around the circle's edge, to make a disk with the spiral on it. Push the toothpick through the disk's center, making sure the stick is a tight fit.

3 Spin the disk like a toy top. One way, the line seems to move inward and disappear into the stick. The other way, it seems to move out and fall off the disk's edge. Of course, it really goes nowhere!

Moving circles

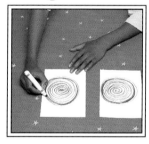

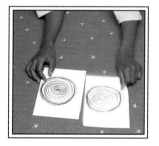

Color wheel

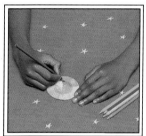

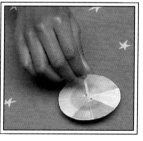

1 For moving circles, draw several sets of spirals or circles on a large white card. Make them clear and colorful. Do the same again, for a second set. Hold one card and move the other in small circles.

2 Can you make sense of what you see? Do the circles seem to rotate? This is a very unusual scene that the brain has trouble understanding. What effect do you see if you move both cards in small circles?

1 For a color wheel, divide a disk of card (4 inches across), into seven equal slices or segments (about 51° each). Color in the segments like a rainbow (the colors of the spectrum), in the correct order: red, orange, yellow, green, blue, indigo, violet.

2 Push a toothpick through the center, and spin fast. The colors merge into white (or perhaps gray). This is because white light is a mixture of many different colors of light: the spectrum. The spinning wheel merges these colors to form white.

EARS AND HEARING

Listen carefully. What can you hear? Even in the quietest place, there are sounds – whistling wind, rustling leaves, singing birds, a car or a plane. Hearing is the body sense that detects sound waves. These are invisible "ripples" that pass out from any object making a noise, whether it is a cat purrrrrrring or a hi-fi pounding out music. The ripples are vibrations, or fast back-and-forth movements, of the tiny floating molecules that make up air. Vibrations pass through air into your ears, which are inside the head, almost behind the eyes.

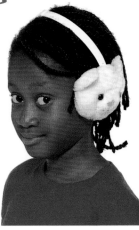

Protect your ears from extreme cold, or too-loud sounds, or very dusty air, with ear muffs. Like eyes, ears are delicate and easily harmed. Never push or poke anything into the ear canal. It should keep itself clean naturally.

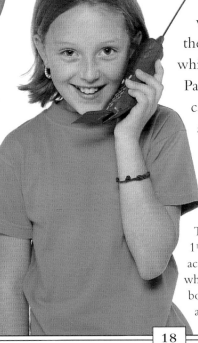

The inner parts of the ears detect the vibrations and change them into nerve signals, which go to the brain. Parts of the inner ears called semicircular canals also help to sense movements and gravity, to help you keep your balance.

Ear shapes
What we call "the ear" has little to do with hearing. It is simply a curved flap of skin and cartilage (gristle) on the side of the head. Ears come in many shapes and sizes, but this has little effect on hearing. They gather sound waves and funnel them into the ear canal.

On the phone
When you listen on the telephone, sound waves go from the earpiece, straight down the outer ear canal. This is the dark hole in the outer ear, and it is about $1\frac{1}{4}$ inches long. At its end is a thin piece of skin stretched across, called the eardrum (shown on the opposite page), which is about the size of your fingernail. The sound waves bounce off the eardrum and make it vibrate, or shake back and forth.

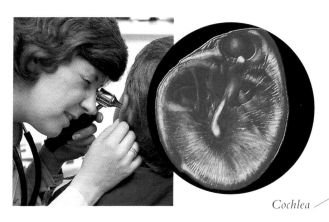

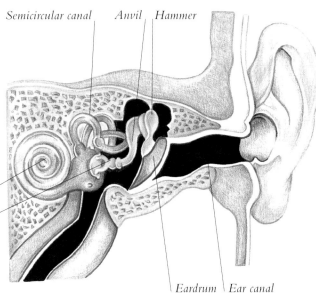

Semicircular canal   Anvil   Hammer

Cochlea

Stirrup

Eardrum   Ear canal

A doctor looks into the ear using an otoscope, to check for infections or other problems. The eardrum looks like a patch of thin reddish skin, with the hammer bone just behind it.

Low and high sounds

Some sounds are deep and booming, like thunder or a big drum. Others are high and shrill, such as a piercing scream or a cymbal. This is called pitch or frequency, and it is measured in Hertz (Hz). Human ears hear many frequencies, from the deepest notes at 25 Hz to extremely high ones at 15,000 Hz. In general, when big objects vibrate, they make deeper sounds. A large hand bell has a lower sound or musical note than a small hand bell. Some animals can hear ultrasounds. These are sounds too high-pitched for our ears to detect, like the squeaks of bats.

Inside the ear

Sound vibrations hit the eardrum and pass along three tiny bones, the hammer, anvil and stirrup, to fluid inside the snail-shaped cochlea. Here the vibrations are turned into nerve signals that go along the cochlear nerve to the brain.

Not too loud

The loudness of a sound is called its volume. It is measured in decibels. Sounds louder than about 85 to 90 decibels can damage the delicate inner parts of the ear, especially if they go on for a long time. So loud earphones or music speakers can harm your hearing. People who work near noisy machines, such as road drills and airplanes, wear earplugs to cut out the sound and protect their hearing.

LOUD AND QUIET

W HEN you hear a very loud noise, like a banging drum, do you turn away and put your hands over your ears? And when you try to hear something very quiet, like a whisper, do you lean forward and turn one ear toward it? Your body's position and movements help you to hear, and to keep your ears from being damaged by loud noises. These projects show how you can make sounds seem louder, and how you can see the vibrations of sound waves. The megaphone shown below is a funnel shape, like an extra-big mouth. It collects sound waves from your voice and makes them spread forward only. It also works the other way around, as an extra-big ear called an ear trumpet, which collects lots of sound waves.

Drums are fun but loud. The harder you hit them, the more the drum head (skin) vibrates, and the noisier it becomes. Bigger drums make lower, deeper bangs.

Whispers are quiet, and usually secret. If there are other sounds, like people talking or music playing, you may have to get very close to the whisperer.

Megaphone

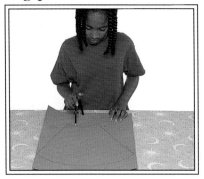

1 Carefully cut out this shape from a large sheet of thin cardboard. When rolled up and taped, it will form a funnel shape, which can be a megaphone or ear trumpet.

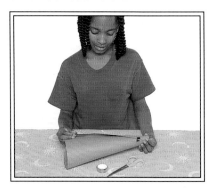

2 Roll the cardboard into a funnel or cone shape. Make the big end as wide as possible, and the small end about 1½ inches across. Tape the cardboard into this shape.

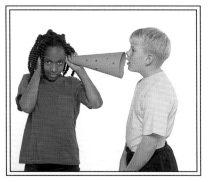

3 Listen normally to your friend talking, then with the funnel as an ear trumpet. Talk to the friend normally, then through the megaphone. Does it help?

Copy your ear

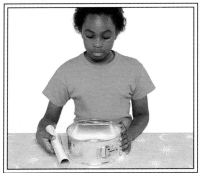

1 Cover one side of the pan with a sheet of plastic wrap. Make sure it is stretched tightly across, with no creases. If necessary, fasten it to the pan with tape.

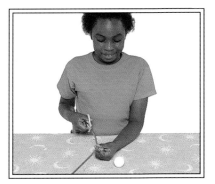

2 Push the short end of one straw into the long end of another. Carefully cut a few slits in the remaining long end so it splays out, ready for the ball.

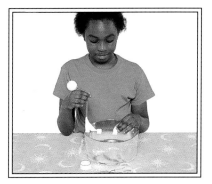

3 Tape the table-tennis ball onto the folded-back slits in the straw. Bend the straws at right angles and secure with tape. Tape the other straw to the plastic wrap as shown.

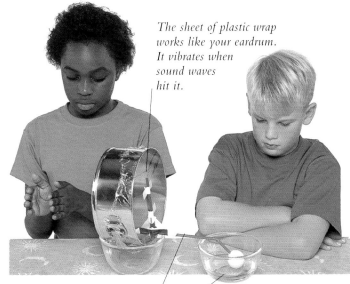

The sheet of plastic wrap works like your eardrum. It vibrates when sound waves hit it.

The straw works like your tiny ear bones. It passes vibrations along to the next part.

The bowl of water is like your cochlea. Vibrations spread as ripples across it.

MATERIALS

You will need: pan without base, like a baking pan, plastic wrap, tape, flexible plastic drinking straws, scissors, table-tennis ball, bowl or dish of water.

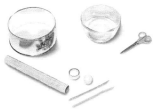

4 Support the baking pan on its side, on another bowl or on some books. Arrange and bend the straws so the table-tennis ball just touches the water in the bowl. This model setup is now like your ear! Make some sound waves near the pan, for example, by clapping. They hit the plastic wrap, which is like your eardrum. This vibrates and sends the vibrations along the straws, which work like the tiny ear bones. The ball makes ripples in the bowl, which is like the fluid-filled cochlea. As a result, you can see sound waves.

NOSE AND SMELL

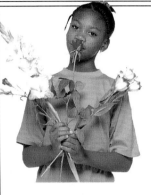

Enjoy the scents of the beautiful blooms. Sniff each type of flower in turn, and ask your friends which scent they like best. People have different personal preferences for scents and odors.

CAN you remember scents and smells for a long time? Perhaps you recall the smell of a holiday beach or the house of a relative. Smell is one of the body's five main senses. The smell area inside the nose detects tiny invisible particles, called odor molecules, floating in the air. Smell checks that our foods and drinks are not bad or rotten. It also warns us of danger, such as the nose-wrinkling smell of soft sinking mud, or the stench of stagnant, polluted water. Smell also gives pleasure, such as the lovely scents of flowers and perfumes and the aromas of good food.

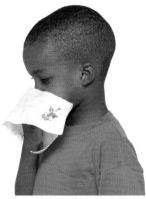

Your nose runs or gets blocked when you have an infection by germs, such as a cold. Get rid of the nasal mucus by sneezing or blowing into a tissue or a handkerchief.

Inside the nose

The nostrils are separated by a dividing wall, the septum. They lead into a large hole called the nasal cavity. When you breathe in, air comes through the nostrils, passes through the nasal cavity, and goes down the back, to the throat and windpipe. The smell area is in the top of the nasal cavity, and it is about the size of your thumbnail.

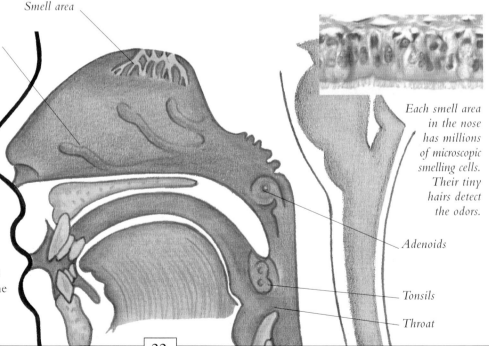

Smell area

Nasal cavity

Each smell area in the nose has millions of microscopic smelling cells. Their tiny hairs detect the odors.

Adenoids

Tonsils

Throat

A mouthwatering meal

Would you eat this well-cooked meal? Smell alone can make you hungry. Your brain recognizes food smells and gets your body ready. Watery saliva (spit) comes into your mouth, ready to moisten the chewing. This is why good foods smell "mouth-watering."

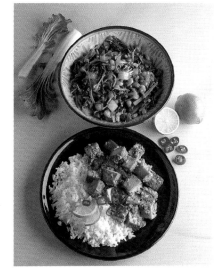

Bad and rotten!

Would you eat this old, rotting food? It looks awful, and if you could smell it, that would be even worse! If foods or drinks smell bad or rotten, they might cause food poisoning, so we avoid them. Smell gives us an early warning before we taste. This is a very important use of the sense of smell.

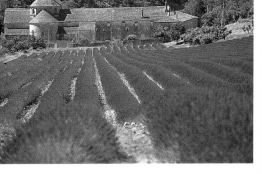

Overpowering fragrance

A few flowers are fine. But a whole field can be overpowering. Some smells are pleasant in normal amounts. But if they are too strong, they are not so nice. The amount or concentration of a smell alters its effects on us.

Sniff, sniff ...

Is that smoke? This odor tells us at once about the risk of danger. The body becomes alert and ready for action. Animals react in the same way to the smell of a forest fire.

FACT BOX

• Most people could identify at least 10,000 different smells, if they had the time to try them all!

• A bloodhound can smell at least 1,000 times better than a person.

• The smell areas inside the top of the nose have 20 million smelling cells.

TONGUE AND TASTE

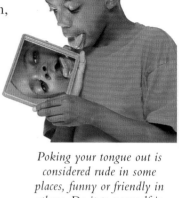

A S you eat your meal, you probably lick your lips slightly to clean them. This also moistens them, so they seal together well and stop food and drink dribbling out. Your tongue does many other jobs, too. It provides your sense of taste by detecting tiny particles called flavor molecules in foods and drinks. With smell, taste helps to tell you if foods are sour, rotten or bad, and should not be eaten. The tongue moves food around in your mouth, so you can chew it all properly. It also helps you to talk clearly, by moving around as you speak and make sounds.

Many animals use their tongues to clean their faces, whiskers, paws and other body parts. People do not need to, since we have hands, soap and water. But sometimes you might lick a stray bit of food or drink from your lips, or even your nose – if you can reach it!

Poking your tongue out is considered rude in some places, funny or friendly in others. Do it to yourself in a mirror. See the tongue's rough surface and the lumps (papillae).

Bumpy tongue

The top surface of the tongue is covered with small lumps and bumps, called papillae. There are different kinds, with larger ones at the back. All the papillae help to grip and rub food as you bite and chew.

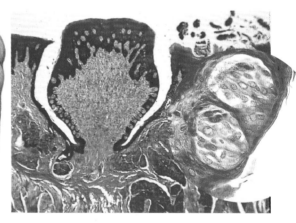

Taste buds

The microscope photograph, above left, shows a cut-through view of one papilla. Set into its lower edges (the stalk) are tiny taste buds. The enlarged view, above right, shows two taste buds with their tasting cells.

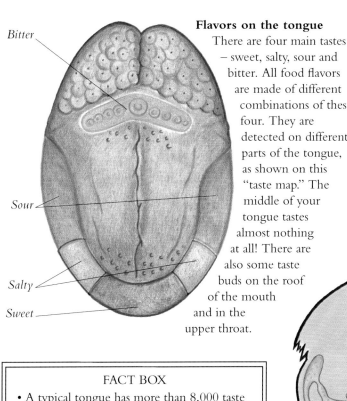

Flavors on the tongue

There are four main tastes – sweet, salty, sour and bitter. All food flavors are made of different combinations of these four. They are detected on different parts of the tongue, as shown on this "taste map." The middle of your tongue tastes almost nothing at all! There are also some taste buds on the roof of the mouth and in the upper throat.

Bitter

Sour

Salty

Sweet

Favorite flavors

Favorite tastes differ from one person to another. Most babies and young people like sweet foods. Some older people prefer salty, spicy or sour tastes. Hardness and texture are also important. Some foods seem slimy, slippery or lumpy. Which of the above foods do you like?

FACT BOX

• A typical tongue has more than 8,000 taste buds on it.

• Each taste bud has 20 to 30 "tasting cells" that detect flavors.

• The tasting cell in a taste bud lives only for 10 days, then it dies. But it is replaced within 12 hours by another one.

• Babies have more taste buds than adults, perhaps as many as 10,000.

• Older people usually have fewer taste buds, perhaps 5,000. So they may say that foods are bland and tasteless, while younger people with more taste buds disagree!

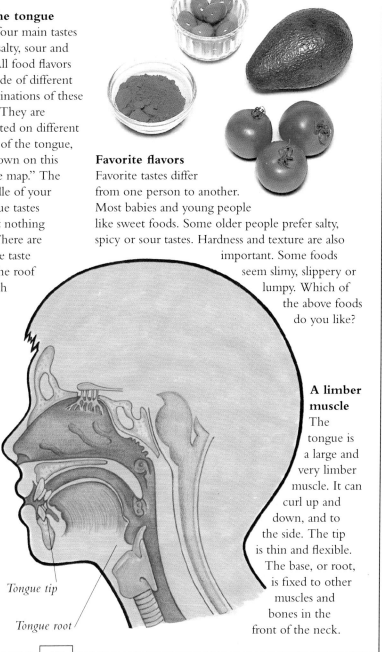

A limber muscle

The tongue is a large and very limber muscle. It can curl up and down, and to the side. The tip is thin and flexible. The base, or root, is fixed to other muscles and bones in the front of the neck.

Tongue tip

Tongue root

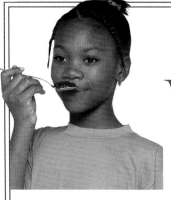

Some smells are similar. Sniff a spoonful of honey, then some jam. Can you tell the difference? They both smell sweet. Perhaps the jam has fruits in it, or the honey has real honeycomb.

SMELL OR TASTE?

WHEN you eat and drink, you use the senses of smell, taste, touch and sight – all together! You detect flavors using the taste buds on your tongue. You detect odors that float from the back of your mouth, up into the back of your nose, as you chew. You assess the temperature, hardness, moistness and texture of food by the different types of touch sensors in your mouth. This is different from taste. You also look at the food with your eyes to get an impression of how it might taste. All four of these senses tell you about the odors and flavors of foods and drinks. But what happens if some of these senses are blocked off? Is it harder to tell what you're eating?

MATERIALS

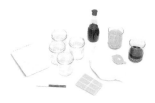

You will need: small pots or jars with lids, cotton, stick-on labels, pencil, notebook, drinks and juices such as apple, orange, grape, tomato, pineapple, coffee, milk and tea.

Sniff test

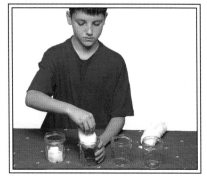

1 Try the sniff test on your friends. Put a lump of cotton into some small jars. Label each one. Make a list in your notebook of which juice or drink you will put into each jar. Keep the list secret!

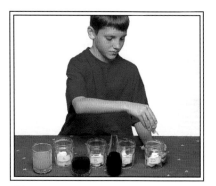

2 Pour onto each lump of cotton the chosen drink or juice. Put on the lids. This stops the smells and odors escaping and mingling together in the air nearby, which could be confusing.

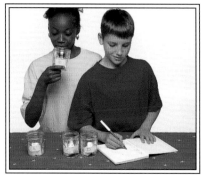

3 Ask your friends to take off the lids and sniff the jars, one by one, without looking inside. The only clue they have is smell. There is no sight, taste or touch. Can they identify what is in each jar?

Taste test

Fading tastes

Why do the first few lollipop licks taste best? If you keep eating the same thing, its taste gradually fades. The flavor molecules are still there, but the tongue becomes less sensitive to them. The same happens with smells. It is called habituation.

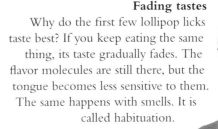

M A T E R I A L S

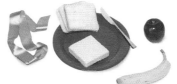

You will need: apple, banana, cheese, bread, pear, melon and similar pale and moist foods, safe knife, blindfold.

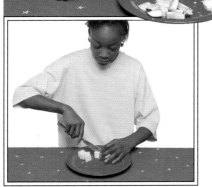

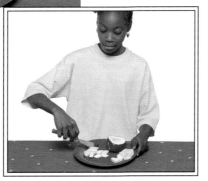

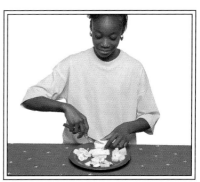

1 Try the taste test on your friends. Carefully peel each food and cut it into small cubes. Try to choose pale-looking foods, so there is little clue in the color. This helps to remove information gained by sight.

2 Cutting the food into cubes also helps to get rid of the clue of shape. This can be detected by sight and also by the touch sensors in the mouth. To make sure, ask the friend to put on a blindfold!

3 When you have cubed all the foods, ask your friend to chew each one a few times, then swallow it. There are hardly any clues from smell or touch. Are the foods easy to identify by taste alone?

NERVES AND BRAIN

Have you used your brain today? Perhaps you have thought hard to solve a problem, or managed to remember something difficult. Thoughts, memories, ideas and wishes all happen in the brain. They are in the form of tiny electrical pulses, called nerve signals. These whiz about among the brain's complicated network of long, thin nerves – millions of them. Much more happens in the brain, too. It is where you feel emotions like love, fear and anger. It is where signals come to, from the senses. It is where you decide to make movements and actions. It is also the control center for all your body's inner processes, like heartbeat, breathing and digesting food. The brain is truly the control center for the whole body.

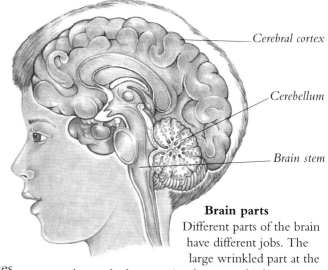

Cerebral cortex

Cerebellum

Brain stem

Brain parts
Different parts of the brain have different jobs. The large wrinkled part at the top, the cerebral cortex, is where you think, remember, decide and become aware of what is happening. The cerebellum at the lower rear makes your movements smooth and coordinated. The lowest part, the brain stem, controls basic life processes like heartbeat.

Safe brain
The brain is very delicate. But it is well protected against knocks by the hard skull bone around it. Even so, it is always wise to wear a safety hat or helmet for extra protection, in case you get a bump on the head.

Seeing the brain
Medical scanners used in hospitals can see inside the head, without any pain or damage (and without cutting it open)! They reveal any injury or disease. This false-color picture shows the wrinkled cerebral cortex and the two eyes with their optic nerves.

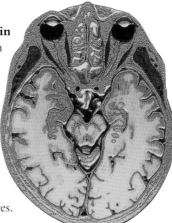

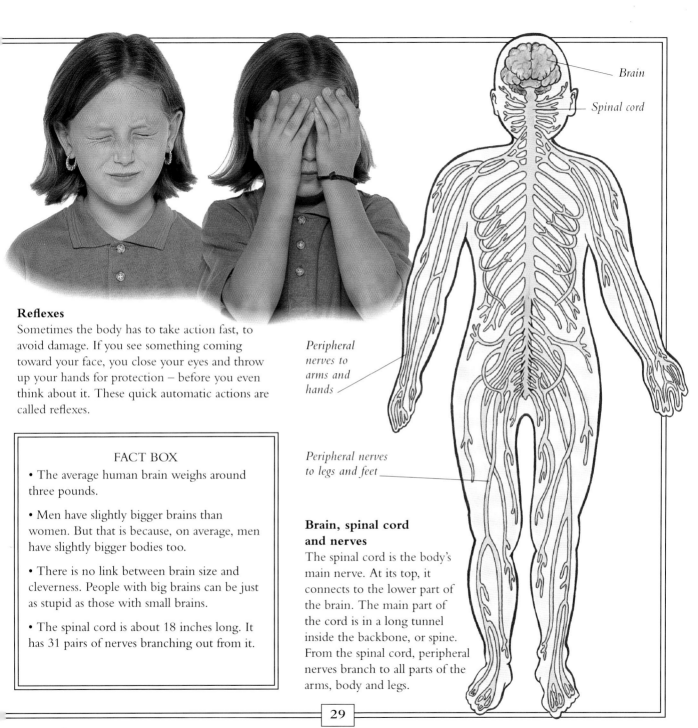

Brain

Spinal cord

Peripheral nerves to arms and hands

Peripheral nerves to legs and feet

Reflexes

Sometimes the body has to take action fast, to avoid damage. If you see something coming toward your face, you close your eyes and throw up your hands for protection – before you even think about it. These quick automatic actions are called reflexes.

FACT BOX

• The average human brain weighs around three pounds.

• Men have slightly bigger brains than women. But that is because, on average, men have slightly bigger bodies too.

• There is no link between brain size and cleverness. People with big brains can be just as stupid as those with small brains.

• The spinal cord is about 18 inches long. It has 31 pairs of nerves branching out from it.

Brain, spinal cord and nerves

The spinal cord is the body's main nerve. At its top, it connects to the lower part of the brain. The main part of the cord is in a long tunnel inside the backbone, or spine. From the spinal cord, peripheral nerves branch to all parts of the arms, body and legs.

AWAKE AND ASLEEP

WHEN you wake up in the morning, and it feels as if you have had a good rest, most of your body has. But some parts, like your heart and lungs, have been working all night. So has your brain. During sleep, it is busy doing various activities. No one knows exactly what, or why. But they must be important, because people who cannot sleep become confused, and suffer headaches and pains. They may even collapse.

When the brain and body need sleep, they tell you by feeling tired. If you ignore this, they go to sleep anyway. Young children can drop off almost anywhere!

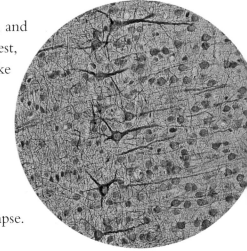

Movement planning center

Movement center

Touch center

Taste center

Other sight centers

Main sight center

Talking center

Hearing center

Smell center (in middle of brain)

Cerebellum for movement coordination

Nerve cells
Like other parts of the body, the brain and nerves are made of cells. They are called nerve cells or neurons. They have long, thin branches that connect to other nerve cells. There are about 100 billion nerve cells in the brain, forming an immense network of pathways for nerve signals.

Brain centers
Different parts of the brain's outer surface, the cerebral cortex, deal with nerve signals coming from the senses. The signals from the eyes arrive at the seeing (visual) center, at the back. They are sorted and compared with patterns of signals already in the brain's memory. In this way, you recognize what you see. Other senses have similar centers.

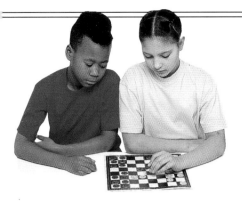

The sides of the brain

The brain looks the same on each side. But the sides have different main activities. The left side takes charge in logic and reasoning, like solving problems in a step-by-step way, working with numbers, writing and speaking words. The right side tends to take the lead in creative and artistic processes like having ideas, recognizing patterns, painting pictures and making music.

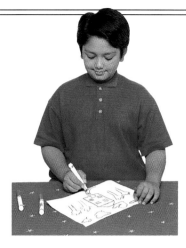

Falling asleep   *REM (dreaming) sleep*   *Waking up*

Deep sleep   *One hour*

Sleep and dreams

When you nod off each night, first you go into deep sleep. Body processes such as heartbeat and breathing slow down, and muscles relax. But after a time, these speed up slightly. Muscles twitch and eyes flick about under closed lids. This is REM (rapid eye movement) sleep, when dreams usually happen. Then you go into deep sleep again, and so on, through the night.

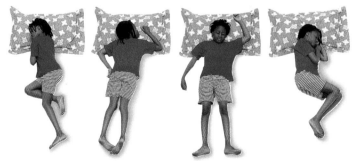

Busy in bed

You do not stay completely still all night. Otherwise you would squash the nerves, blood vessels and other body parts you are lying on. You move and shift your position as many as 50 times.

FACT BOX
• A newborn baby needs about 20 hours of sleep each day.

• A 10-year-old needs about 10 hours' sleep each night.

• An adult needs seven to eight hours' sleep each night.

• But these are all averages. Some people have less sleep, others more. But whatever your sleep needs are, don't fight them.

MEMORIES

THERE is not one place in the brain for memories. They seem to be spread through several brain parts. Memories are probably complicated connections and pathways for nerve signals among the brain's millions of nerve cells. There are two stages to making a memory. One is to remember, which is to store the information in your brain. The other is to recall it, which is to find it again. You can play a sport or musical instrument better with practice – and you can do the same with memories. The more you try and learn to remember, the better you should become. There are also a few memory aids, short-cuts and "tricks" that you can use, as shown here.

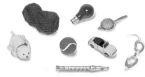

MATERIALS

You will need for the memory tray: a selection of household toys, ornaments, utensils and similar small items.

Some people write about their lives in a diary. This is a memory aid. They can look up a day which happened long ago. From a few words in the diary, they can begin to recall many other things that happened. The few words act as a memory trigger.

Memory test

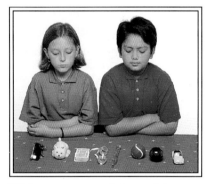

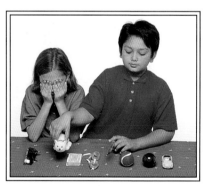

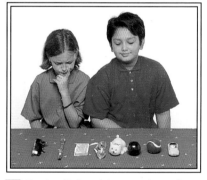

1 Lay out a row of about eight or ten small and everyday objects on a table. A friend looks at them for about 20 seconds. He or she tries to remember their names and their positions in the row.

2 The friend closes eyes, and you move two objects, to swap their positions. The friend then looks again, and tries to identify the moved items. This is usually easier than remembering all the items in order.

3 Study all the objects again and try to memorize them. One trick is to make a word from the first letter of each of their names. Or try to include their names in a silly story, which makes them easier to recall.